-To Grace
"So that others may live."

Towards the end of my first year in practice, I was blessed to offer healing to a little girl in the last two weeks of her life. During those last two weeks, thanks to her family's dedication, she was able to play pain-free without the heavy medication she had been on during the years of clinical trials she had undergone. Months later, on my knees in the sorrow of this great loss, I cried out in total surrender, "Why had this sweet little girl been taken?"

In a split second, I felt the greatest peace and joy beyond words, I saw a horizon of clouds and a single point of light from which all things expand out. From there I looked down and saw good and bad swirling together to create an experience here on Earth. Although, the pain of loss was not dampened, I also knew the need my mother and I had to finish creating this text and to deliver it to all those on their sacred journey from dis-ease to de-light.

Having seen the many disease processes affecting humanity and the lifestyle changes required to upgrade the body, mind and spirit, one has to ask, if all of our symptoms and our losses are somehow leading us back to the garden?

In the military town that I was in at the time, there is a motto that represents the love and diligence of the people, "So that others may live." May those of us who remain behind, be brave enough and have faith enough to know that a greater plan is underway. And, may we always speak and act in alliance with what we know in our hearts to be true.

Rhiannon

A special thank you to Sheila Spence for editing and tilling the soil with her hands to feed the people from the garden!

And, to Natalie Gonder for photography and for reminding us all to be as little children!

Table of Contents

What's Your Why?...	3
How This Book Works...	4
Preface...	6
How Methionine Restriction Works...	8
Proportions...	61
Meal Plans...	63
Grocery List...	66
Introduction...	68
From Scratch...	73
Sprouting...	77
Dehydration...	78
Breakfast...	80
Sauces...	90
Sides, Snacks & Appetizers...	99
Entrees...	112
Salad Dressings...	133
Soups & Salads...	135
Baked Goods...	148
Desserts...	156
Drinks...	163
Calculations Addendum...	165
Low Methionine Food List...	169
Research...	190

Cure For The Garden: Featuring The Methionine Restriction Protocol   Copyright 2019. DocRhi.com

What's Your Why?

When I (Rhiannon) graduated with my dual graduate degree in chiropractic and eastern medicine, I was flying high! I was my class valedictorian and had successfully published my thesis. Then came the bad news...

I'd had been diagnosed with cancer. Me! A healthy 31 year-old! How could this be?

My mom, a soils microbial ecologist and herbalist, quickly began researching natural cancer treatments when she came across a diet with **over 40 years of research** in successfully shrinking tumors and reversing all kinds of other diseases.

So **how come other doctors weren't talking** about it? And, why didn't we learn about it in one of the number of nutrition classes we'd taken? It was being dismissed by researchers as being too hard to follow. We thought, "You wouldn't eat fruits, vegetables, legumes, and seeds to save your life!" Well if no one else is going to do this diet, we are!

So we spent the next several years transitioning our diets and trying out all kinds of recipes and strange exotic foods that we went all over the place to find, and finally honed in on **the simplest, yummiest, and most comforting foods** on The Methionine Restriction Protocol, using foods you can easily find.

Our hope for the world is that we will all transition to this diet, saving our own health and the health of the planet. And, that no child will ever pass on before their time due to preventable diseases again.

Cia & Rhiannon, Mother and Daughter

This diet has over 40 years of research showing amazing effects in:

- **Shrinking Tumors**

- **Extending Lifespan**

- **Burning Fat Faster by Resetting Metabolism**

- **Correcting Metabolic Diseases such as Diabetes High Blood Pressure and High Triglycerides**

- **Resolving and Attenuating Autoimmune Issues**

- **Reducing Anxiety and Depression while Improving Focus and Memory**

- **Helping to Alleviate Pain Inflammation**

Your Why Must Extend Beyond Yourself

Cure For The Garden: Featuring The Methionine Restriction Protocol

How This Book Works

In the following pages, we will go over:

- **Why and how the Methionine Restriction Protocol works**
- **What you eat**
- **How to prepare your mind and your kitchen for optimal success**
- **How lifestyle can empower your transformation**

When I, Cia (Doc Rhi's Mom) started my trek toward eating this way, I had no idea that this diet was already laid out for me thousands of years ago, that thousands of journal articles were already written on it, and that it would align with my goals as an environmental scientist to help heal the planet. When I started eating this way, I was intuitively listening to a body suffering from chronic fatigue, extreme pain from polyneuritis and chronic flu-like symptoms that placed me in bed with my eyes closed for nearly four whole months.

No books, no movies or TV, no phone calls, I didn't have the energy. I couldn't keep my eyes open. I just laid in my bed trying to relax because the more I relaxed, the less I hurt. Doctors diagnosed me with polyneuritis. I had never heard of it and neither had anyone else. Since I didn't have cancer or anything thought of as life threatening, I was left to fend for myself without any treatment other than the option of pain killers.

Doctors didn't know how I got polyneuritis or how to get rid of it. Fortunately for me, the pain medication merely made my head foggy and my body nauseous. The pain didn't dim even slightly. I had to find my body's way out of the mess. Today, I share how I healed with you. This book is **the place in my journey where I am inviting all of my sisters and brothers to join me on this path toward the beautiful, powerful bodies we were made to have**. Even if you have tried every diet known to man, this is the protocol that will not only remodel your body for optimal health but can transform the health of the planet as well.

We will be truly healthy only when our home is healthy too.

Let's jump right in!

Preface

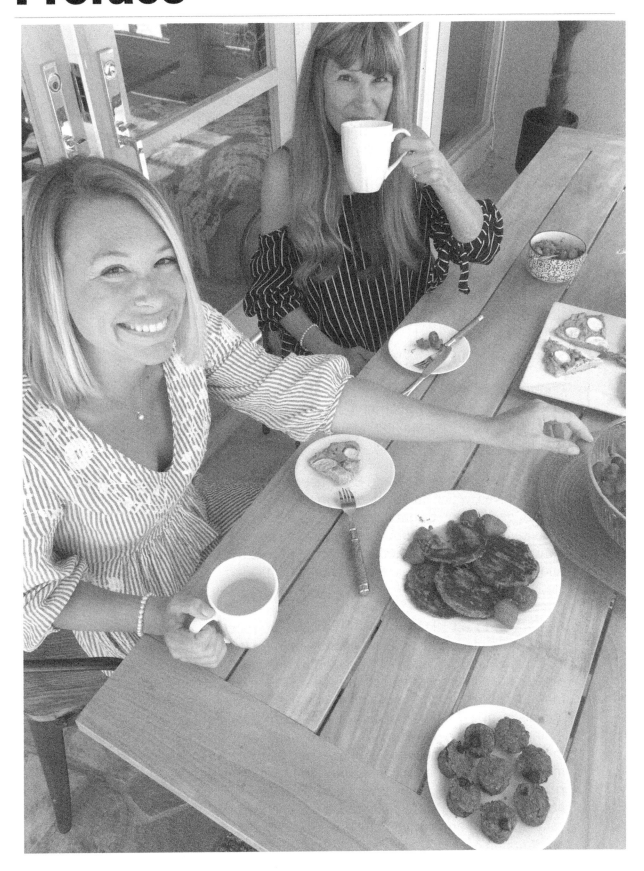

Cure For The Garden: Featuring The Methionine Restriction Protocol

Tips For Getting Started

When you begin exploring the art of cooking, it is a good idea to try to recognize flavors. Each time that you add a spice, taste the dish you are making. When you go out to a restaurant, try to guess which spices were used and ask the chef if you are right. Chefs love it when patrons are into the artistic side of food. In Eastern nutrition, it is considered important to eat warm, cooked or fermented foods because it is easier to absorb their nutrients. But, you can also add warming spices such as cinnamon and ginger for the same purpose!

If you would like to cook with frozen food instead of fresh that's fine. Frozen produce is generally less expensive and can have more plant-nutrients, or phytonutrients, because it is generally vine-ripened and flash-frozen instead of picked early. They cook in about the same amount of time as fresh, just don't add any water as they have a tendency to make their own as they cook.

Carefully read the ingredients of everything! Our food labeling system is set up for the benefit of the food producers not the consumers! Make sure you check that there are no added sugars, grains, animal products and preservatives. Sometimes, anti-oxidant rich vitamins such as A, C, and E are used as preservatives, which can be healthy in small quantities. You don't want to overload your body with any vitamin. When in doubt, if you know you are eating the vitamin, don't add a vitamin supplement and check with your physician. The majority of vitamins are better absorbed through our food anyway.

> *Hippocrates cautioned us, "Let your food be your medicine, and your medicine be your food."*

Remember to eat all the colors of the rainbow. Yellow squashes, as well as other winter squashes, can help with pain reduction. This is just one example of how our food can help us stay healthy. Each color brings different healing properties to our meals. Dr. James Duke of the U.S.D.A., formerly of Purdue University and one of the country's best phyto-chemists says; "An old-fashioned vegetable soup, without any enhancement, is a more powerful anti carcinogen than any known medicine." And, Hippocrates cautioned us; "Let your food be your medicine, and your medicine be your food." Eating every color of vegetable, each day, helps to make sure we get all we need. Spices also help, so learning to spice your food is not only yummy, but spices add color, diversity, antioxidants and other critical phyto-chemicals (plant nutrients) to our diets.

Cure For The Garden: Featuring The Methionine Restriction Protocol   Copyright 2019. DocRhi.com

The Best Diet For You, Is The Best For Earth Too

Preface

You are only as healthy as the environment you live in.

By the 1920's, J. Russell Smith and his fellows at University of Pennsylvania knew that food forests were the only way to sustain our crops and the world. The Japanese knew it even earlier!

Trees stop the loss of soil with their roots. They hold the water in the surrounding soil by slowing the run off and allowing the time for the rain to soak in. And, they release fresh, clean air. Trees can even suck up toxins and excess salt to create a pristine environment. Trees open up their pores to add moisture to the atmosphere to create a small area or micro-climate that is better able to sustain other trees, which create more of a micro-climate, and so on. Trees, welcome other plants to their neighborhoods. A forest creates a sustainable future for the earth and everyone on it! There are some great studies that have been conducted on what is called, permaculture. Or, sowing layered forests with plants that can flourish in the local geographic area if they are planted in a certain order. We urge you to do your own research on this topic, YouTube is a great place to start!

In order of the closest to the sky, to the nearest to the ground, these layers are:

- **The tallest trees like pines and cedars**

- **Trees that form a canopy to shade**

- **Understory of shaded trees, shrubs, ferns & vines**

- **Shaded nursery plants and herbs**

- **Mushrooms and roots**

A forest is not only made up of trees. 5 separate layers make up a forest. We get **different foods from these different layers.**

Although, there are different definitions of the layers for forests in different parts of the world, you can see that each layer gives us a plethora of foods and medicines. From pine nuts and apples to mustard greens, truffles and potatoes, the forests of our world offer everything we need to maintain optimum health.

A forest is the only sustainable agriculture! So cook from this cookbook to use all of the layers and consider growing your own food forest!

Cure For The Garden: Featuring The Methionine Restriction Protocol   Copyright 2019. DocRhi.com

What Do You Want From Your Food?

What do you want from your food? we've asked this question many times and almost always got the same answers.

- I want it to be simple, quick and travel well.

- I want delicious, healthy food.

- I don't want to have to plan and prepare things, I just want food when I want food.

- I want my food to not have any calories.

- I want my food to feel good and make me feel better when I am down.

- I want my food to be cheap.

What if you found food that was naturally packaged for travel and ready when you are ready to eat?

What if you found food that was delicious and healthy?

What if you could cut your grocery bills?

What if you could eat as much as you wanted without gaining weight, in fact much of it would help burn calories?

What if you found food that could reduce your pain and help you to be more flexible and move easier?

What if your food helped you to detoxify and could keep your heart young?

What if your food could truly and we mean really, keep you young and could guard your body from cancer? What if you found out that your food could actually shrink tumors and could be used even if chronic conditions are already in your life?

What if your food could change how your DNA to make you healthier?

Dr. James Duke of the U.S.D.A., says "An old-fashioned vegetable soup, without any enhancement, is a more powerful anti carcinogen than any known medicine."

Cure For The Garden: Featuring The Methionine Restriction Protocol   Copyright 2019. DocRhi.com

Ancient Indications

Sound too good to be true?

It's not!

What if we told you The Methionine Restriction Protocol was described in ancient texts thousands of years ago?

The Book of Genesis, also called The Tanakh, written between 2500-3000 years ago, says, "Behold, I have given you every herb bearing seed, which is upon the face of all the earth, **and every tree, in the which is the fruit of a tree yielding seed; to you it shall be for meat."**

What does this include?

Let's look a little closer for the answer. The next verses state, "And the earth brought forth grass, and herb yielding seed after his kind, and the tree yielding fruit, whose seed was in itself, after his kind."

Comparing the two verses, you can see something has been left out from the second verse describing what was created versus the first verse which defines our food. That something is the tender grasses. Tender grasses are the grasses or what we call grains. They are called 'mono,' meaning one, and 'cot,' meaning leaf, because they grow from one leaf into stalks or blades. These are corn, wheat, rye and other grasses and grains. We were not intended to eat much grain! It turns out, grains contain an amino acid, which if limited allows tumors shrink and helps our bodies to heal from metabolic diseases including diabetes, high blood pressure, cardiopulmonary issues and others. It can even be used in advanced chronic diseases safely with doctor's or lab testing. Grains are not ideal for our bodies or for the earth. As we have already mentioned, grain crops are not the best crops for sustainable agriculture.

Okay, so we don't eat grains, so what do we eat?

During fasting times **in the Hindu tradition, which is believed to be at least 2800 years old, grains are switched out for water chestnut flour which is almost completely methionine free!** We've included this amazing flour in many of our recipes! It can be found at Indian markets or online. In this text, we will show you many ways you can eat traditional foods with healthy substitutions that even taste better.

Cure For The Garden: Featuring The Methionine Restriction Protocol   Copyright 2019. DocRhi.com

Your Search Stops Here

So why haven't we heard about this diet before?

Chances are you have learned about parts of the Methionine Restriction Protocol but thought it wasn't for you.

We are not going to lie to you!

Food is like our mother, we run back to what we know and love for comfort. Unfortunately, not all parents are good for us and neither are all the diets we grew up loving. Some diets cause pain, obesity and disease. Running back to unhealthy food is like running back to an abusive parent. It is what we know, love and feel comfortable with.

If you are interested in **vigor and beauty**.

If you want to be **healthy and happy**.

If you are looking for a way to **prolong your life** and the lives of your family, this may be your path.

But how can we go without bread?

Simple, quick bread recipes are included in this book along with other tricks and tips to make your changes and substitutions easy, fast and healthier.

So what are you waiting for? Are you afraid that you will have to give up your ice cream or you cookies?

Is learning to eat for vigorous health too time consuming or too much of a hassle?

What if we told you not to change anything until after you finish this book?

In fact, we don't think you should change anything until you have finished every word!

Then, if you still think it is not worth the effort and the changes to protect your health and the health of your family, don't change one thing!

Cure For The Garden: Featuring The Methionine Restriction Protocol   Copyright 2019. DocRhi.com

So how do you do it?

However, if you are looking for a way to stay younger and healthier. If you are searching for the path to lose weight, chronic disease and depression. If you never again want to look for a new diet, this is the protocol·pointed out to us as long ago as the book of Genesis was written and is backed by today's best science.

The Methionine Restriction Protocol is the last diet you will ever need!

Still think you could never give up cheese or meat? What if you found out that **there is a fruit that tastes like blue cheese** or **an unripe fruit that when prepared correctly looks, chews, and tastes like meat**? And, it isn't soy or gluten based. They are fruits! The Methionine Restriction Protocol was made for us. It respects all life and preserves it for future generations without depleting the soil or deforesting our planet. And, all this without breaking the bank

So how do you do it?

The first part of this book is how and why the Methionine Restriction Protocol works.

Then we explain what you will be eating.

We've filled this book with tricks and tips to make the substitutions and changes easy.

We have also shared the little things you can do to make this **the last book you will ever need to read about a diet protocol**.

If you are ready to achieve vibrant, youthful health, lose weight, and even lose depression, let's get started, but remember don't make these changes until you have finished this short book to the last word!

Cure For The Garden: Featuring The Methionine Restriction Protocol   Copyright 2019. DocRhi.com

Dispelling Myths About Diet

Let's start by dispelling some of the myths we are taught about diet.

Scientists know how to stop the obesity epidemic in this country.

They know how diet can shrink tumors and cause mutated cells to commit suicide to stop cancer before it starts. The first studies based on the Methionine Restriction Protocol began in 1974. Yes, that's right. Scientists have known about this since 1974! The diet was administered as a laboratory mixture of nutrients without methionine, not with real food. The problem scientists found with this diet, according to many journal articles, is that finding palatable foods are too difficult to enable people to adhere to this diet. Seriously? You can't eat fruits and vegetables to save your life? Come on!

Some scientists (not all) are incredibly smart people **paid by the corporations that bring you packaged, processed foods and dyed meats**. If corporations can sell foods in a packaged, processed form, they call it added value. This is because they can take inexpensive produce, process it and get a much higher price for it. They win because they get more money, they have extended the shelf life of many of the products, no longer need to worry about getting the produce to the market fresh and ripe. The Methionine Restriction Protocol ensures fresh produce is in your diet with **all the phytochemicals, enzymes, antioxidants and nutrients brought to you packaged by nature.**

Methionine is called an "essential" amino acid, meaning it is allegedly essential to our diet because we can not make it. **It is now known that methionine is made by our body from homocysteine. So, it is not an essential amino acid**. In fact, when homocysteine is not converted into methionine in our body, the homocysteine builds up and becomes toxic, leading to chronic disease.

Cure For The Garden: Featuring The Methionine Restriction Protocol

Scientific Data And Research

What does science say about The Methionine Restriction Protocol?

The National Institutes of Health says, "This diet will make it feasible to extend life without restricting calories." The protocol is built around the restriction of one amino acid, methionine. Methionine is one building block for proteins. But don't worry, it's a protein that needs to be minimized for optimal health. **You will still consume more than enough healthy proteins.**

Methionine restriction **decreases a process called oxidation which keeps our telomeres (the protective caps on our chromosomes) healthy.** This increases the life of our cells so we can have greater human longevity and vitality! Have you ever wondered why the people in Genesis were reported to have lived so long or even if the reports were true? Well, this may be one of the reasons for their long lives.

The Methionine Restriction Protocol is not only great for humans, it is great for the environment too! The Methionine Restriction Protocol will push big agriculture to grow more fruit, nut and legume trees and less mono-cultured field crops because no grains, or what was referred to as "tender grasses," are eaten. No mono-crops are needed to feed livestock either. The soil isn't plowed so we aren't going to lose top soil or cut down more trees to plant more fields. Sustainable tree forests with the fruits of trees, shrubs, vines, roots and undergrowth will continuously provide all the food necessary to live long healthy lives. **Franklin D. Roosevelt once said, " A nation that destroys its soil destroys itself. Forests are the lungs of the land, purifying the air and giving fresh strength to our people."**

> *The National Institutes of Health says, "This diet will make it feasible to extend life without restricting calories."*

How Methionine Restriction Works

People At Risk Of Heart Disease

Only 1 in 25 people diagnosed with a life-threatening condition, follow their doctor's instructions to change their diet and lifestyle.

Margaret Mead once said, "It is easier to change a man's religion than to change his diet."

The Methionine Restriction Protocol is **for those that are sick of being sick** or want to help to save the life of someone they love.

The Methionine Restriction Protocol can help to reduce the risk of heart disease and stroke.

According to the Center for Disease Control and U.S. Department of Health & Human Services, about 1.5 million people die from heart disease and stroke in the U.S. every year. This is 1 in every 3 deaths, most of which were preventable with diet and lifestyle changes. More than 525,000 people each year have their first heart attack and 210,000 have their second.

Their SECOND HEART ATTACK! And, most are preventable!

Who are the **people at higher risk for heart disease**? People with:

- Diabetes
- High blood pressure
- High cholesterol
- Obesity and adiposity
- Poor Diet
- Physical inactivity

The above are all symptoms of metabolic imbalances.

The Methionine Restriction Protocol can help to **bring your body back into balance and reverse metabolic syndrome by actively fighting obesity and stopping the critical causes of inflammation by remodeling our cells.**

Cure For The Garden: Featuring The Methionine Restriction Protocol   Copyright 2019. DocRhi.com

Health And Wealth

1 in every 6 dollars spent on medical care is spent on cardiovascular disease. Heart disease and stroke alone costs the nation an estimated **$316.6 billion dollars in health care costs and lost productivity**, and this statistic is from 2011! People we know have **lost their homes, their retirements and their dreams of travel** due to the healthcare costs attached to chronic disease. The Methionine Restriction Protocol can empower your health and help to guard your dreams.

According to the National Cancer Institute, 1,685,210 people in 2016 will be diagnosed with cancer. That is 448.7 per 100,000 men and women each year and 168.5 of those 100,000 men and women will die of cancer each year.

39 percent of the men and women in the U.S. will be diagnosed with cancer during their lifetime. Science demonstrates much of this is not necessary. **We can take control of our health and our genetic switches!**

The National Institutes of Health project cancer costs to reach at least $158 billion by the year 2020! And, it could reach as high as $207 billion according to the National Cancer Institute. This is not necessary!

"The first wealth is health."-Ralph Waldo Emerson

The Methionine Restriction Protocol is for those wanting to claim longevity, vibrant health and keep their money to spend on things they want! As Ralph Waldo Emerson stated, "The first wealth is health."

So if you are ready to start healing yourself naturally and stop spending as much on pharmaceuticals this protocol can help you to **start transforming your cells within days**. If practiced continuously for 6 months, some medications can be discontinued completely with the help of your primary care physician.

Cure For The Garden: Featuring The Methionine Restriction Protocol

How Methionine Restriction Works

Are You Ready To Slow Down The Aging Process?

Do you want to be one of the 25% of people willing to change your lifestyle to give yourself amazing health?

In 2015, the National Institute of Health published a review from a workshop held in Italy, asking if we were ready to slow aging in humans. They agreed there is **sufficient evidence demonstrating safe interventions to delay aging and increase healthy lifespan in humans** by preventing disease onset for many chronic conditions. This workshop took place in 2013!

So why are we still suffering from these chronic conditions when these represent **the greatest financial burdens and challenges** in both the developed and developing countries?

This book will equip you with the vital information to live longer, healthier, happier lives!

Studies have shown the Methionine Restriction Protocol can help:

> *"There is sufficient evidence demonstrating safe interventions to delay aging and increase healthy lifespan in humans" -NIH Workshop, 2015*

- **shrink tumors and cause cancer cells to commit suicide** by starving them of the component cancer needs but your cells do not

- **extend lifespan** by lowering free radicals, oxidative stress, and lengthening telomeres

- **burn fat faster** by increasing mitochondria (cell powerhouses) to raise your metabolism

- **correct metabolic diseases such as diabetes, high blood pressure and high triglycerides** by increasing your sensitivity to insulin and decreasing bad fats like triglycerides and free fatty acids

- **resolve and attenuate autoimmune issues** by stepping down inflammation messengers (histones)

- **reduce anxiety and depression while improving focus and memory** by slowing norepinephrine (stress neurotransmitter) pathways

- **help alleviate pain and inflammation** by reducing oxidative stress

Cure For The Garden: Featuring The Methionine Restriction Protocol

How Methionine Restriction Works

Take Control Of Your Health And Happiness

The Methionine Restriction Protocol is for anyone that wants to take control of their own health and happiness and help their friends and loved ones too!

If you want to slow down aging, reduce pain, inflammation and cancer risk, lose weight and keep it off, have more energy, and be vitally healthy and happy, the Methionine Restriction Protocol is for you!

How does the Methionine Restriction Protocol do this?

It does all this by ensuring we get all the phytochemicals, nutrients and antioxidants we need while restricting acidity, free radicals, oxidative stress and methionine. When we restrict methionine, it changes how our body uses our food, forcing an increase in mitochondria (cell powerhouses) and insulin sensitivity.

The Methionine Restriction Protocol is naturally very high in all of the things we need. The Methionine Restriction Protocol, when practiced correctly, is naturally low in calories and unwanted fats so **you can eat more and still lose fat, and decrease depression, pain and inflammation**. Decreasing dietary methionine causes a detoxification of the toxin, homocysteine and slows down pathways that increase the stress neurotransmitter, norepinephrine. This helps to protect us from anxiety and insomnia to help ensure happiness as well as healthiness! Although some of the reasons this diet works are still being uncovered, the phytochemicals found in foods eaten on The Methionine Restriction Protocol can help us to utilize our DNA properly to build the factors, enzymes and proteins we need to be healthy and happy. The protocol stops oxidative damage, protects us from mutations and also helps diseased, mutated cells to commit suicide to ensure they don't become cancerous. All we need to do is adhere to what we were told to eat by the ancients.

Cure For The Garden: Featuring The Methionine Restriction Protocol   Copyright 2019. DocRhi.com

Getting Enough Protein And B12

Do we have to worry about getting enough protein?

Most people eating a western diet eat too much protein! This can lead to gout, kidney disease and other disorders. When you eat according to the Methionine Restriction Protocol, you are getting foods that are naturally low in Methionine but still have other amino acids necessary to continue to construct, maintain and repair our bodies. If you eat fruits, vegetables, legumes, nuts and seeds, you will receive all of the proteins you need and still maintain low methionine.

The only things you need to think about when correctly practicing the Methionine Restriction Protocol is eating enough foods with B12 and Vitamin D, and only if you have a preexisting issue. B12 deficiency is very rare in healthy individuals.

B12 and iron are found in sea vegetables like purple nori and in vegetables grown in organically fertilized soil. Organic fertilizers are high in vitamin B12 and in the form that is most easily absorbed by our bodies. Chemical fertilizers do not supply vitamin B12. This is one of the many reasons to eat organically grown fruits and vegetables or even grow your own. The Methionine Restriction Protocol is **naturally higher in folate, vitamins and antioxidants.**

Cure For The Garden: Featuring The Methionine Restriction Protocol   Copyright 2019. DocRhi.com

Vitamin D And Genetic Problems

Too much protein isn't good for our bodies. It can lead to a buildup of uric acid, toxins and pain. Some people have trouble metabolizing protein and its building blocks. If you have an **MTHFR gene substitution (nick-named the Mother-Father Gene)**, cysteine metabolism issues, or trouble flushing homocysteine out of your system (ask your doctor for lab tests), incorrect diet can result in a toxic buildup of homocysteine. You may need a vitamin B12 supplement whether you use the Methionine Restriction Protocol, or not. Studies have shown vitamin B9 (folate), from leafy greens, beans and nuts, and the nutrient called betaine, from beets and other plant sources, can lower homocysteine concentration without the need for increased vitamin B12! With this protocol you can eat all of the vegetables you want to get plenty of folic acid betaine and keep toxic homocysteine levels down.

Sometimes babies are born with a genetic problem of the **MAT1A gene** that predisposes them to toxin buildup. Usually, these children develop severe nervous system problems. Cases have been published, showing that strict dietary methionine restriction can prevent these neurological deteriorations so that physical growth and psychomotor development can be completely normal despite the genetic condition!

"Put your mushrooms in a windowsill for some sun before eating them."

Vitamin D is found in mushrooms and sunlight. Put your mushrooms in a windowsill for some sun before eating them. They collect vitamin D for you. To collect your own vitamin D, make sure you get out in the sun every day before 11 am or after 3 pm without sunscreen. Twenty minutes is good for light skinned people if you have darker skin, you may need more. We naturally make our own vitamin D and getting out in the sunlight in the morning resets our body clocks, converting melatonin into serotonin and back, enabling us to sleep and be happy! Americans only spend 03% of their time outdoors. **To ensure ample vitamin D be sure to get outside daily.**

Cure For The Garden: Featuring The Methionine Restriction Protocol   Copyright 2019. DocRhi.com

Even More Vitamins

Choline is important to cell membrane health and can also be transformed into betaine. **Choline is naturally found in peanuts, spinach, cauliflower, soy, lentils and flax seeds**. These are all foods eaten in the Methionine Restriction Protocol! Choline, betaine and B vitamins help transform homocysteine into methionine. Getting rid of homocysteine is really essential to our health because it is a toxic intermediate. It can build up in our system and cause disease and pain. Eating the correct foods can aid in the transformation of homocysteine and get it out of our systems. This aids in the normal methylation of our DNA.

Methylating our DNA is like hanging little magnets on it. These little methyl magnets are made of a carbon and hydrogen. These magnets can change the shape of our DNA, and regulate where and when our DNA is copied to make our proteins and other factors that keep us healthy. The correct methylation of our DNA enables the proper copying and building of amino acids, proteins and other factors we need to run our bodies and maintain our health. Some of these factors can keep mutated cells from becoming cancerous. But when too much methylation occurs, it is called hypermethylation and can suppress the genes that help us fight cancer. So having the correct methylation, as The Methionine Restriction Protocol ensures, is very important.

Fiber, B12 And Leaky Gut

The Methionine Restriction Protocol provides a rich supply of dietary fibers, which **welcome the friendly bacteria** found in our intestine. Vitamin B12 is produced by specific bacteria, the Methionine Restriction Protocol can provide the correct environment for vitamin B12 producers to grow and multiply, to help supply vitamin B12 to the body. Fermented foods including **soy tempeh contain vitamin B12, as do dried shiitake mushrooms and a fermented black tea** called Bata Bata-cha.

B12 deficiency rarely occurs in healthy people. Vitamin B12 is reabsorbed with our bile into the liver from our intestine, so it is reused over and over. Again, ask your doctor to help you to decide if you need a supplement.

Building Healthy Intestinal Microbes

The bacteria inside of our Gastrointestinal tract is called our microbiome. Their role in our health is not yet completely understood. What we do know is without correct, friendly bacteria, we don't make the products needed to maintain healthy. Incorrect microbiomes have been linked to vitamin **B12 malabsorption, Crohn's, colon cancer, anxiety and depression, and even hot flashes and osteoporosis.** The Methionine Restriction Protocol helps us to fertilize our internal gardens and grow friendly, happy bacteria in our guts to help maintain health and happiness. When our intestinal brain, called our enteric nervous system, tells us we feel bad, it can be our **friendly microbes sending messages through the cells of our Vagus nerve**. Our Vagus nerve helps us to stay in a state where we can rest, digest and heal, with our stress nervous system offline. Happy, healthy microbes in our food means a happy, healthy body!

You may have heard of Leaky-Gut Syndrome, when the junctions between your intestinal cells lose their tightness and undigested food and other non-food particles leak into the body. Leaky-Gut is connected with inflammation, cancer and early aging. Restricting methionine can help to protect against Leaky-Gut as well as build-up of many toxins in the digestive tract, such as sulfites, glutamate and homocysteine. This is important because toxins such as glutamate can cause stress hormones to rise leading to nerve damage, anxiety and insomnia.

Cure For The Garden: Featuring The Methionine Restriction Protocol

What If I Have A Chronic Disease

What if we or someone we love is already chronically ill, can we use the Methionine Restriction Protocol?

Yes. Methionine Restriction has been shown in studies to improve quality and prolong life and, in many cases, to reverse and prevent diseases.

One Italian study, found the Methionine Restriction Protocol to be beneficial to in kidney disease, even advanced cases. They found it was safe when used with doctor's care. The study showed, it **cuts down on the frequency of dialysis and slows further loss of kidney function**, by reducing protein intake and decreasing the nitrogen load on the kidneys.

If you already battle with metabolic disorders such as diabetes, high blood pressure and high cholesterol and triglycerides, the Methionine Restriction Protocol is a safe, effective way to alleviate and **overcome not just the symptoms but the causes** of the disorders and bring your body back into greater balance.

"One Italian study, found Methionine Restriction to be beneficial to in kidney disease, even advanced cases."

The Methionine Restriction Protocol shrinks tumors and causes cancer cells to commit suicide, while stopping many DNA mutations. This is achieved **through epigenetic changes to our DNA.** Epigenetics is the study of changes in gene function so that we are not destined to have the same diseases as our family. Methionine Restriction also **reduces oxidation and reactive oxygen species, increases the alkalinity of our pH and increases antioxidants to help fight cancers.** Many phytochemicals found in plant-based diets even have the same effects as chemotherapy but are much safer.

Cure For The Garden: Featuring The Methionine Restriction Protocol   Copyright 2019. DocRhi.com

Enhancing Your Metabolism

How does the Methionine Restriction Protocol enhance metabolism?

Like we've said, The Methionine Restriction Protocol restricts the "essential" amino acid, methionine. This causes our cells to use other, more calorie expensive pathways to make the things our bodies need like energy or ATP. Increasing energy expenditure, raises calorie use and turns on fat burning! This limits fat storage and limits adiposity. In short, we lose weight. Because we are not storing fat, we are not becoming obese. If we are not obese, we also don't acquire the diseases of obesity such as insulin resistance, disordered fat metabolism and inflammation.

When a person has insulin resistance, they cannot process sugar correctly. It also turns off fat burning. **However, dietary methionine restriction can actually help to reverse insulin resistance. This means if you are looking at losing a limb or your eyesight due to diabetes, don't hesitate, jump now.** The Methionine Restriction Protocol, when practiced properly, enhances insulin sensitivity and metabolic flexibility. Specifically, it increases the adipocyte (fat cell forming) hormone, adiponectin and the liver hormone fibroblast growth factor 21 to

"Studies show it can even give you a more youthful metabolism!

decrease belly fat and improve how you use sugar. Methionine restriction produces a significant reduction in fasting insulin and blood glucose. One study says it can even give you a more youthful metabolism! It may do this by remodeling your DNA to turn on the fat burning and heat producing capacity of white fat making it more like the brown fat that babies have to burn more calories!

Don't forget, if you have a chronic disease, find a compassionate doctor to oversee your lab tests and progress. You will need to remember to evaluate and monitor your pharmaceuticals, especially insulin and blood pressure medications while changing your diet, weight and metabolism.

Losing Weight

Why does the Methionine Restriction Protocol help you to lose weight?

Methionine restriction doesn't only turn on decrease the accumulation of new fat cells, because of the increased energy expenditure it causes you to burn more calories. Technically, the decrease of methionine causes an us to release protons (energy packets) as heat in our cells' mitochondria (the power house of the cell). This makes our food, or calorie-to-energy ration less efficient. In other words, it takes more food to make the energy we use. **So, we can eat all we want of the right foods and The Methionine Restriction Protocol revs up our metabolism.** This means you can eat the right foods and still lose weight!. Often, when symptoms of metabolic syndrome are found in a person, their fat burning is completely turned off. The Methionine Restriction Protocol turns fat burning back on raising your metabolism!

This is of paramount importance because obesity is linked to the development of so many chronic diseases such as:

- Hypertension
- Type 2 Diabetes
- Atherosclerosis
- Heart Disease
- Cancer
- Inflammation and chronic pain

The Methionine Restriction Protocol is less energy dense and can result in reduction in calorie intake. Although less calorie dense, it is very high in nutrient density. It is packed with phyto-nutrients, antioxidants and other factors that support a healthy body, mind and even DNA.

The bottom line is you can eat more of the correct foods, lose weight and build a happier, healthier, more beautiful body.

How Methionine Restriction Works

Your Immune System

How does the Methionine Restriction Protocol support our immune system?

The Methionine Restriction Protocol can help keep the boundaries or "tight junctions" of our digestive tract intact and tight. Whereas, consuming animal proteins and grains can result in increased permeability in the tight junctions of our digestive system. This causes "leaky gut syndrome". **Leaky gut can allow the movement of bacteria and undigested proteins into the blood stream.** Once in the blood stream, these invaders can adhere to organs and tissues where our immune system soldiers sniff them out and try to attack them. This causes us to attack our own tissues and organs leading to certain autoimmune disorders. Without the constant bombardment of additional proteins, the immune soldiers, known as macrophages, can clean up the invaders and relax. This decreases inflammation and the discomfort that is sometime related to it.

When cooking with beans, we recommend pressure cooking or sprouting them to reduce the lignans, the nutrient in beans which can be difficult for those with gastrointestinal deficiency to digest.

The Methionine Restriction Protocol contains phytochemicals known to be antibacterial, antifungal and antimicrobial. These little soldiers help to keep us health and step down inflammation at the same time. Because plants can't run away from invaders, they are experts at making phytochemicals to fight them. We can gain their strength by adding them to our diets.

How Methionine Restriction Works

Cure For The Garden: Featuring The Methionine Restriction Protocol   Copyright 2019. DocRhi.com

Decreasing Inflammation And Pain

How does the Methionine Restriction Protocol decrease pain and inflammation?

Because the Methionine Restriction Protocol reduces obesity, inflammation is reduced. This occurs because fat cells manufacture their own hormones and factors that increase inflammation. In addition, **methionine restriction causes a far greater reduction in the genes that start the inflammatory cascade.** It is thought that the reducing of chronic inflammatory states like obesity, diabetes and cardiovascular disease is the reason for the increase in longevity with methionine restriction but, some studies also suggest these delays in aging are due to other reasons as well. At times, merely the loss of weight can benefit joints such as the hips and knees by decreasing the pain involved with arthritis from heavy weight bearing.

As previously discussed, Choline, found in many of the Methionine Restriction Protocol foods like soy, cauliflower, lentils and flax seed, have demonstrated anti-inflammatory properties in studies conducted on inflammatory arthritis. It decreases reactive oxygen species (the cause of oxidation that occurs in inflammation and cancer) and suppresses inflammatory responses. Choline can also transform to **betaine, which is useful in transforming toxic homocysteine into methionine.** High levels of homocysteine are linked to inflammation, pain and even neuro–degenerative disorders.

The foods of the Methionine Restriction Protocol lack fats containing arachidonic acid, which is pro-inflammatory. "Pro" means they cause inflammation and pain. The foods in the Methionine Restriction Protocol also lack purines that breakdown into uric acid. A buildup of uric acid can accumulate in the joints and can cause pain and inflammation. This is known as gout and eating meat and eggs can cause it. In a clinical study of 40 participants from Michigan State University, 6 weeks of a whole-food plant-based diet demonstrated significant improvement in energy and movement in people suffering osteoarthritis or degenerative arthritis. **The American Dietetic Association recognizes whole-food, plant-based diets to be beneficial in the prevention and treatment of rheumatoid arthritis and osteoarthritis.** 12 months of a gluten-free whole-food, plant-based diet showed decreased pain.

Cure For The Garden: Featuring The Methionine Restriction Protocol   Copyright 2019. DocRhi.com

Decreasing Inflammation And Pain

Studies have shown reduced pain in as little as two weeks with dietary methionine restriction.

The reason for the decreased pain is thought to be decreased inflammatory proteins and arachidonic acid. Nonsteroidal anti-inflammatory drugs work by limiting the metabolism of arachidonic acid. So, you will no longer need to take over the counter pain killers if you keep your intake of arachidonic acid low with this protocol. The Methionine Restriction Protocol dramatically reduces the availability of the precursors used to make these painful proinflammatory prostaglandins.

If you are sensitive to gluten, your body treats it as a foreign invader and attacks, causing inflammation and pain. The Methionine Restriction Protocol contains no grains and therefore, no gluten. Dairy products can also lead to inflammation causing gastrointestinal pain and bloating. No dairy is eaten on the Methionine Restriction Protocol.

Remember to expand to eating all colors of fruits and vegetables- "Yellow squash helps with pain reduction!"

Chemicals such as artificial sweeteners, monosodium glutamate and others, cause headaches and inflammation due to a buildup of toxins and our bodies' inability to filter them properly.
The foods included in the Methionine Restriction Protocol, particularly fruits and vegetables, contain natural products called phytochemicals that can aid in the biotransformation of toxins like polychlorinated biphenyl and others. Easting all colors of fruits and vegetables gives us a wide array of phytochemicals to combat toxins. But, the affects of phytochemicals are biphasic, meaning, a certain amount is beneficial to the body but too much may overload the liver and cause toxicity. This is one of the reasons phytochemicals should be ingested in our diet and monitored very closely if given in supplement form.

Cure For The Garden: Featuring The Methionine Restriction Protocol   Copyright 2019. DocRhi.com

Inflammation, Pain And Bone Health

Eating foods on The Methionine Restriction Protocol provides a higher ratio of omega-3 essential fatty acids to omega-6 fatty acids to help alleviate pain. The Methionine Restriction Protocol contains nuts and the fatty acids from nuts are high in the anti-inflammatory Omega 3 fatty acids, monounsaturated fatty acids, is low in saturated fats with zero bad trans-fats. Mono-unsaturated fats are named "mono" meaning one, because they only have one double bond that can oxidize and cause inflammation. So, if you are going to add fats to your food, like in salad dressing, make sure it is a monounsaturated fat such as olive oil.

The Methionine Restriction Protocol can help you to have more anti-inflammatory Omega-3 fatty acids than taking a fish oil supplement. Why is this so important? Because inflammation causes not only pain, but other chronic organ problems. Studies on the Blue Zones, the areas where people live the longest such as the California Seventh-day Adventists, demonstrate high associations between ischemic heart disease in men eating beef three times per week when compared to vegetarians. They also found significant protective associations between eating nuts at least five times per week in both men and women. The risk of ischemic heart disease was 31% lower over a lifetime in those that ate nuts and 37% lower in male vegetarians compared to non-vegetarians.

We have pain receptors that are turned on by acidity. **Acidity can also lead to osteoporosis (bone loss), which is a painful degeneration of our bones.** Acidity can also allow unwelcome microorganisms into our bodies leading to disease and pain. The Methionine Restriction Protocol keeps the pH of our bodies balanced through the ingestion of alkaline and pH neutral vegetables and fruits, turning off pain, protecting our bones and keeping our microorganisms friendly.

In addition to decreasing osteoporosis by maintaining a more alkaline pH balance, foods on The Methionine Restriction diet have been shown to increase bone toughness and flexibility. The digestive health caused by eating restricted methionine also allows for the correct amount of the hormone, serotonin to be produced. If this hormone is not regulated by a happy digestive system, osteoporosis can occur.

Cure For The Garden: Featuring The Methionine Restriction Protocol   Copyright 2019. DocRhi.com

Shrinking Tumors To Fight Cancer

We already know that restricting methionine in our diet reduces inflammation and free radical damage to cells. But did you know that it can help to prevent cancer, shrink tumors and increase cancer treatment success? The Methionine Restriction Protocol can help to prevent cancer, even if you are genetically inclined towards certain types. Cancers can be formed due to toxic interactions with such things as plastics, cosmetics, pesticides, smoked foods and smog. But, methionine restriction can stop cancer cell reproduction because without methionine, they can't methylate (a process involved in building proteins). Studies show that reducing methionine can cause tumor cell death without hurting normal, healthy cells.

It even shrinks tumors in studies conducted on mammals and in cell experiments by reducing the amount of cancer stem cells, slowing the rate of the cancer to make new cells and causing tumor apoptosis (cell death). Many cancers are completely dependent on methionine to form, such as those that develop from viruses. So, if you don't eat methionine, the cancer can't eat it either.

Dietary methionine restriction is safe and may used concurrently with standard treatment methods. In fact, because methionine restriction lowers glutathione levels in tumors, it may make tumors even more responsive to treatments with chemotherapy and radiation. In cases where a person already has cancer, we highly recommend seeking individualized consultation with a Methionine Restriction Protocol Coach to calculate methionine levels and determine a proper fasting schedule as well as individualized supplementation.

Cure For The Garden: Featuring The Methionine Restriction Protocol   Copyright 2019. DocRhi.com

Reducing Cardiovascular Disease

Why does the Methionine Restriction Protocol reduce cardiovascular disease?

The Methionine Restriction Protocol significantly decreases the pro-inflammatory messengers that cause inflammation and it remodels our cells so we can handle oxidative stress better. When we have oxidative stress in our blood stream it roughs up the lining of our blood vessels, called atherosclerosis, literally blood vessel scarring. This scarring causes narrowing of the vessel and causes dangerous clots to form. This protocol can help to dissolve dangerous clots and help to resolve cardiovascular disease.

Additionally, dietary methionine restriction increases fat burning and fat storage in the liver in particular. This lowers the fats circulating in your blood stream, and limits fat being deposited in the walls of arteries.

The healthy fats included in the Methionine Restriction Protocol come from sources such as olives, avocado, pumpkin seeds, walnuts and other nuts, leafy greens like kale, squashes and root vegetables. These fats are mostly monounsaturated fatty acids. Monosaturated fatty acids are good fats that protect the body from oxidation and damage due to reactive oxygen species.

The Methionine Restriction Protocol also offers foods containing a-linolenic acids (ALA), which can prevent coronary heart disease. Increased ALA reduces the risk of myocardial infarction and fatal ischemic heart disease even if the patient smokes. Don't get me wrong, smoking still puts you at greater risk!. The ALA eaten from plant sources can convert to other healthy fats called DHA and EPA in small amounts. Purslane, a common weed that we highly recommend using as a salad green contains trace amounts of DHA and EPA as well as ALA. Walnut, avocado, almonds, flax and olive contain ALA and only small amounts of omega-6 fatty acids. This balances our fatty acids and enables us to convert our fats as needed.

Cure For The Garden: Featuring The Methionine Restriction Protocol

Reducing Cardiovascular Disease

A correct balance of omega-3 fatty acids and omega-6 fatty acid helps many body functions including:

- Lowering cholesterol levels and balancing fat synthesis

- Reducing triglyceride levels

- Aiding digestive secretions,

- Aiding respiratory muscle contractions

- Reducing inflammation, helping our immune system and reducing cancer.

- Aiding our nervous systems and moods

- Preventing formation of blood clots, reducing their breaking off and causing heart attacks or strokes.

Animal foods contain the saturated fats that are linked to cardiovascular disease. **Studies from Harvard and the Cleveland Clinic demonstrate that heart disease can be reversed by diet.**

Additionally, we would like to address some of the other reasons to use plant based foods. **As an animal eats, he or she accumulates the toxins included in their foods.** For instance, if a large fish eats many small fish, the large fish accumulates all of the toxins the small fish stored in their bodies. This is called bio-accumulation. Our environment is continually getting more polluted and the animals are storing more and more toxins, as are we. One way to cut the toxins going into our bodies is to eat organic plants that are grown in safe places. Some plants are even purposefully used as bio-accumulators, to clean up mine tailings and superfund (toxic dump) sites. We must be careful our foods are grown safely, in clean areas and avoid eating bioaccumulating animals and plants.

Cure For The Garden: Featuring The Methionine Restriction Protocol

Reducing Cardiovascular Disease

As we have stated, The Methionine Restriction Protocol mostly uses **unheated mono-unsaturated oils that are added after cooking your food.** Heating oils can easily cause them to break down and become toxic to the body. Cold pressed, non-chemically derived oils are full of healthful bioactive, phytochemicals because they aren't heated or pH altered with any other chemicals. The phenolic compounds found in olive oil have antioxidant capacities that make them potent free radical scavengers. These powerful phenolics help stop bad fats from oxidating and fight thrombosis, or blood clot formation. It is no wonder, in the 2000 year old story of the good Samaritan, he uses olive oil to bind the wounds of an injured man. Olive oil decreases cancer cell growth, division and migration. Olive oil also helps prevent organ fibrosis and is important to anti-aging of organs. Extra virgin olive oil can induce epigenetic changes in how our DNA is copied to help prevent the genes associated with aging from being switched on.

"Extra virgin olive oil can induce epigenetic changes in how our DNA is copied to help prevent the genes associated with aging from being switched on."

The vegetables eaten in the Methionine Restriction Protocol contain sulfur and, together with sunlight, can help to prevent cardiovascular disease, atherosclerotic plaque buildup and damage through oxidation. This protocol can protect us from oxidative damage, inflammation and even necrosis or tissue death.

The mucopolysaccharides, or long chain sugars, found in plant foods such as **yams, plantain, aloe vera, mallows, sea weeds and many seeds, help repair damaged epithelial tissues, like those found in our blood vessels and skin.** This helps to help keep our organs and skin healthy and youthful.

Cure For The Garden: Featuring The Methionine Restriction Protocol — Copyright 2019. DocRhi.com

Youthfulness And Longevity

Besides the phenolics and mucopolysaccharides mentioned above, how does the Methionine Restriction Protocol keep us young?

Scientists used to think that the only way to extend lifespan was through caloric restriction, or reducing the amount of food you ate to very little. Now, evidence shows that this protocol has the same effects as a calorie restriction diet except **you don't have to restrict your calories!** Calorie restriction diets are well known to prolong life and increase health and wellbeing. The Methionine Restriction Protocol can do this while allowing normal amounts of food to be eaten. The calories eaten on The Methionine Restriction Protocol are incredibly high in nutrients and phytochemicals needed to maintain and repair the body. And, methionine restriction may be able to actually **reverse the negative effects of aging caused by yearly weight gain, obesity, insulin resistance, and cellular oxidative stress**.

It also reduces the accumulation of genetically damaged cells to increase the longevity of our cells, tissues and organs. Like the calorie restriction diet, the Methionine Restriction Protocol can protect our cells from oxidation damage, heavy metal stress and other toxicity.

Restricting the amount of methionine you consume also **decreases the breakdown of telomeres, which are the protective caps on our chromosomes**. Telomere length is one of the most predictive markers of aging ever discovered. They keep our cells from breaking down and dying.

When you eat the proper foods to restrict methionine, the building blocks of triglycerides are limited. This decreases fatty deposits and lipogenesis (fat creation) in the liver, keeping your liver healthy and young.

The Methionine Restriction Protocol can also increase longevity through epigenetic mechanisms on the gene called FGF21. Expression of this gene in the liver, and glucose balance, helps the body to run more efficiently and avoid age related metabolic diseases. **This not only increases longevity, it also increases quality of life with lasting health and happiness.**

Without health, we have nothing!

Cure For The Garden: Featuring The Methionine Restriction Protocol   Copyright 2019. DocRhi.com

How Methionine Restriction Works

Mood, Memory And Focus

How does the Methionine Restriction Protocol reduce depression, anxiety, and memory and attention problems?

The brain consumes huge amounts of energy and oxygen, and it produces tons of free radicals. Worst of all, because the brain is full of fats, our nerves are is especially vulnerable to oxidative damage. The oxidative stress of free radical damage leads to depression, anxiety, and other neurodegenerative and psychological disorders, such as Alzheimer's and Schizophrenia. The Methionine Restriction Protocol **aids brain functioning and communication by flooding our bodies with antioxidants and fatty acids to control oxidative stress**.

When we use our food to make energy in the powerhouse of our cells, called mitochondria, we generate free radicals. Because these **free radicals are missing electrons, they run around trying to pull electrons from other places**. This stealing of electrons causes a domino effect, where the free radical pulls the first electron off the second, and the second pulls it off the third and this continues until an antioxidants comes and stops this process by sharing an electron. An ample amount of antioxidants from our food are necessary to stop free radicals from causing mutations and other damage by stealing electrons.

The Methionine Restriction Protocol decreases reactive oxygen species and free radicals, and increases antioxidant mechanisms to limit oxidative stress. It does this by lowering the fats that are susceptible to oxidative stress and increasing the amount of antioxidants in our body.

Reactive oxygen species aren't all bad! They are used as weapons against invaders. Unfortunately, when there isn't enough phytochemical antioxidants to stop them, the free radicals change proteins, DNA and lipids and alter cellular functions.

Higher cognitive skills such as good decision making and being able to delay gratification is linked to the thickness of the part of our brain called the cerebral cortex. Poor nutrition can lead to degeneration and thinning of this part of the brain causing memory, focus and other cognitive problems. **Studies conducted specifically on Alzheimer's and methionine restriction show that lowered methionine is linked to a decrease in the plaques causing brain degeneration!**

Cure For The Garden: Featuring The Methionine Restriction Protocol

How Methionine Restriction Works

Mood, Memory And Focus

Stopping oxidative stress with antioxidants and cell remodeling can help to stop oxidative damage leading to:

- Panic disorders
- Post-traumatic stress disorder
- Obsessive-compulsive disorder
- General anxiety

Phytochemicals found in a plant-based diet can increase the enzymes necessary in the parts of the brain called the hippocampus, amygdala and cortex to prevent anxiety. We all know we can't think straight when we are stressed. The food we eat can stress our brains and bodies or it can make us healthier and happier. The Methionine Restriction Protocol can also help balance the genetic expression of neurotransmitters and other factors that aid memory and cognitive processes. Specific foods have higher amounts of these neurotransmitters, such as **serotonin found in plantain, pineapple, banana, kiwi, plum and tomatoes, melatonin in fenugreek spice and mustard, and tryptophan in peanuts, beans and potatoes.**

The phytochemicals in the foods of the Methionine Restriction Protocol suppress pro-inflammatory factors to help stop inflammation which can damage mood areas of the brain. **Antioxidant modulation of oxidative stress can even benefit schizophrenia and bipolar disorder.**

Additionally, higher levels of B vitamins as well as vitamin C, D,E and omega-3 fatty acids have been linked to brain health and can decrease the rate of brain shrinking that happens as we age.

How Methionine Restriction Works

Cure For The Garden: Featuring The Methionine Restriction Protocol   Copyright 2019. DocRhi.com

What Stops Us From Changing

So why isn't everyone using this protocol?

The researchers in clinical studies say that the reason dietary methionine restriction isn't used is because it is too difficult to follow and people will always cheat.

When we read this, we knew we had to develop this protocol to help people everywhere make the changes necessary for healing.

Research has demonstrated only about 25% of people given a life-threatening diagnosis actually change their diets and lifestyles.

When we asked people why they don't here are some of the answers we got back:

It is too difficult to cook for myself.

I don't have the time or the energy.

The thought of changing my diet makes me really emotional, teary and feel out of control.

I don't know how to change.

Why bother? I am going to die anyway.

I don't want to give up the little pleasures.

Changing my diet never worked before. Why should it now?

"It is easier to change a man's religion than to change his diet."

-Margaret Mead

When we developed this protocol, we took all of these reasons into consideration and, over several years, developed recipes that are comforting, creamy and make our taste buds and our hearts contented. We also studied new research on tools for changing that we call Brain-Training. We teach Brain-Training our online workshops for The Methionine Restriction Protocol, as well as, offer a coaching certification because we learned that **the best way to stay on a lifestyle coarse is to teach it to others.**

Cure For The Garden: Featuring The Methionine Restriction Protocol   Copyright 2019. DocRhi.com

Food Addiction

This is food addiction talking!

The changes in dopamine and serotonin levels due to cravings and satisfaction of those cravings are **the same as levels seen in cocaine addiction and in alcoholism**. In fact, the combination of high fats, sugars and salt is **more addicting than cocaine**. With one added caveat, we need to eat!

When you place addictive foods in your mouth, you are continuing an addiction that could lead to disease, pain, mutilation and death. We all already know this. There is no need to remind or upset you. Eating while upset can lead to more addictive eating as well!

What if we told you, we can give you the information to transform your life? We use a special technique we developed to go along with the diet portion of this protocol called, Brain-Training to help overcome food addictions. You can go to www.DocRhi.com to find our courses on Brain-Training.

What if you could still satisfy the cravings and stay true to healthy eating?

What if there is a way to connect with others that are transforming their lives and diets?

What if you had the support you needed to start a healthier, happier lifestyle? Connect with us on Facebook at The Methionine Restriction Protocol.

How ready are you to manifest vibrant health and happiness in your life and the lives of your loved ones?

Supplemental Reading

Because we don't want this to read like a research paper, We have added a list of journal articles for you to look up at the end of this book. If you want more detailed information about the science behind the Methionine Restriction Protocol, please follow your curiosity! More and more findings are demonstrating the efficacy of eating this way. Go ahead and prove it to yourself.

Cure For The Garden: Featuring The Methionine Restriction Protocol   Copyright 2019. DocRhi.com

Embodying Vibrant Health And Happiness

What can we do to embody vibrant health and happiness?

Change depends, not on the selection of one food, but on the consistent and continuous selection of beneficial foods on a daily basis. This book offers suggestions on how to plan your diet and lifestyle to enhance your energy both physically and mentally to bring amazing benefits!

This means if you are adding beneficial foods to your diet daily, avoiding problem foods and substituting unhealthy foods for healthy foods, you are winning! There is no failing, only giving up. The only failure is to stop reaching for health and happiness.

If you have too much fat around your waist, high blood pressure, high blood glucose, abnormal lipid levels, and increased fatigue and irritability, you can benefit from the Methionine Restriction Protocol! Every small change you make is a step towards a longer healthier life. The Methionine Restriction Protocol can help to rebalance your metabolism to avoid chronic diseases and rapid aging caused by inflammation. The American Diabetes Association recommends a focus on plant based sources such as lentils and beans for protein intake, a focus on healthy fats, avoiding saturated animal fats and trans-fats. They also suggest spacing out your meals throughout the day and moderation of salt intake. The Methionine Restriction Protocol helps with this and more. We invite you to use this book as a guide towards incredible health.

Are you ready for true transformation?

The Science Of Prevention

If you choose the Methionine Restriction Protocol daily, you can avoid:

- **Over-using your cell's insulin** receptors (the little gates that welcome and lets insulin escort glucose into your cells).

- **Over-taxing your pancreas** (it tries to make more insulin to escort because glucose isn't being let in and stays at high levels in the blood).

- **Obesity and new storage of fat** cells (fat burning is ramped up due to derailing of part of our energy making equipment).

- **Cholesterol filled cells** depositing on the inner wall of blood vessels causing inflammation, which damages the lining of blood vessels causing a thickening called **atherosclerosis** (a fatty fibrous growth made of white blood cells lipids, which hardens and contributes to the blocking of blood vessels). This can cause high blood pressure, heart disease and even blood clots.

- **Painful inflammation** caused by oxidation, lack of antioxidants and build up of toxins. Inflammation is the major cause of cancers and autoimmune diseases.

Using The List of Low Methionine Foods

We already know all of the dangers, let's get to the proverbial "meat and potatoes", without the meat of course.

What can we eat?

At the end of this text is a list of over 1000 foods with their methionine quantity. Methionine content is listed per 100 grams of the food. We have taken the time to convert everything to volume (cup) measurements because we never weigh our food but we know what a cup of something looks like. Foods are listed in ascending order of Methionine (less to more). So, if you eat foods at the top of the list, you can eat practically nonstop and never go over the amount of methionine needed each day. The high methionine foods at the bottom of the list must be used as condiments and as additions to other foods in order to limit the grams of methionine eaten.

If you are still wondering about the foods you are used to eating, the ones that satisfy your craving, here is the deal.

Corporations hire professionals to make their foods more addictive by combining fats, salt, and sugars with flavorings. This is why Oreo cookies, fast food burgers and fries are so addicting!

You can combine fats, salt and sugars! But, now you are going to do it with fruits and vegetables! Combining dates, sea salt, nuts or beans, cocoa or carob, and coconut gives you an amazing natural candy to eat (See Desserts). You can eat one a day because you still want to restrict your methionine intake. You can eat ice cream too, Invest in a Yo-nana machine or a good food processor, and use frozen fruit and a little almond milk and vanilla.. And Voila! You have substitutes for addictive foods to help with your transition.

Cure For The Garden: Featuring The Methionine Restriction Protocol   Copyright 2019. DocRhi.com

Methionine Restriction Calculations

Remember, you can eat all the fruits and vegetables you want as long as you limit the grams of methionine consumed each day.

How many grams of methionine can we eat each day on the Methionine Restriction Protocol?

The Recommended Dietary Allowance (RDA) for methionine for adults 19mg/Kg/day. That is 19 milligrams of methionine for every Kilogram of body weight for each day.

When studies restricted methionine to 15mg/kg/day, metabolic balance was restored and additional fat storage was halted. Weight loss was the same as vegan diets but loss of fat cells was higher with the methionine restriction. This means you lose more fat but can keep your muscle! **Studies show an 80% restriction is necessary to achieve the results of anti cancer, anti inflammation and anti aging.**

"Studies demonstrate restricting methionine to 80%of the RDA, shrinks tumors, lowers oxidation and inflammation. An 80% restriction of the RDA is 3.8 mg of Methionine for every kilogram of body weight each day.

Successful methionine restriction diet studies allowed 2mg/kg weight/day to be eaten. This is quite low but after 16 weeks on the diet, no adverse symptoms occurred. Using methionine restriction stops metabolic syndrome in its tracks, can help to reverse pain, diseases and anxiety and does not cause adverse affects on the body.

Other studies demonstrate efficacy at an 80% restriction to shrink tumors, lower oxidation and inflammation. An 80% restriction of the RDA of 19 mg/kg/day is 20% or 0.2 * 19 mg= **3.8 mg for every kilogram of body weight each day.**

***Make sure you are working with a doctor to monitor your biomarkers while on this protocol, as well as monitoring any pharmaceutical drug quantities that may need to be changed as your body begins to work more effectively from your improved nutrition.**

Cure For The Garden: Featuring The Methionine Restriction Protocol   Copyright 2019. DocRhi.com

Methionine Restriction Calculations

The amount of methionine you can eat each day depends on what you want as your perfect weight and how badly you need to reverse metabolic problems and inflammation. The less methionine you consume, the more results you will be able to measure. Studies have demonstrated 15mg per kilogram of body weight will allow changes in fat burning and metabolic balance. However, if you are looking at life threatening conditions or if you are really interested in results, use the calculations below.

At this point, we want to let you know, **you don't need to develop an aptitude for math** to use the Methionine Restriction Protocol, you just need to eat from the top of the food list at the end of this book and you will see results. If all else fails, **remember fruits, vegetables, beans, then a few seeds and nuts!** The recipes in the cookbook are made to be comforting and delicious while achieving low levels of dietary methionine.

If you want precise measurements for maximum results, stick to the lowest quantity of methionine used in research studies which is **2mg for every kilogram of body weight each day, or 8.4mg per pound.**

To proceed with exact calculations yourself, head to the examples in the addendum of this text, or look for a Methionine Restriction Protocol Coach to do the calculations for your specific health goals and needs.

"If you want precise measurements for maximum results, stick to the lowest quantity of methionine used in research studies which is 2mg of methionine each day for every kilogram you weigh. This is 8.4mg per pound you weigh."

How Methionine Restriction Works

Cure For The Garden: Featuring The Methionine Restriction Protocol   Copyright 2019. DocRhi.com

Methionine Restriction Calculations

So now, let's look at the Methionine Content Food List found at the end of this book to see what the woman who want to weigh 120lbs. can eat.

Please note, the unit found on the food chart is grams of methionine per 100 grams of each food.

So what can a 120 lb. woman eat each day?

If we use the 3.8mg of methionine per kilo of body weight per day, a woman who wants to fight chronic disease and wants to weigh 120lbs., can eat 0.206g methionine/day. (If you want to know how this is calculated, see the Addendum.)

0.206g of methionine a day means **you can eat 103 medium sized apples and still not go over the amount of methionine allowed in your diet.**

Or you can eat over...

- 40 cups of unsweetened applesauce,

- or 70 cups of dehydrated mung bean noodles,

- or 200 celery stalks,

- or 16 cups of vegetable juice,

- or 10 cups of squash,

- or 14 cups of snap beans,

- or 10 cups of plantain,

- or 12 cups of olives,

- or 11 cups of blueberries,

- or7 cups of yams,

- or 400 grapes,

- or 3 medium baked potatoes,

- or 2 cups of avocado,

- or 5 cups of raw broccoli,

- or 1 cup of cooked lentils,

Cure For The Garden: Featuring The Methionine Restriction Protocol   Copyright 2019. DocRhi.com

Methionine Restriction Calculations

- or 1 cup of hummus,

- or 8 oz of firm tofu,

- or 3/4 cup of roasted almonds,

- or less than 1/2 cup of dry roasted peanuts or 1/3 cup of peanut butter.

So as you can see, eating enough food to keep full and satiated isn't a problem.

The idea is to keep your methionine low while eating a rainbow of nutrients, phytochemicals and antioxidants, not to eat 100 apples.

Basically, the more methionine in a food, the less of that food you eat in a day. In the Appendix of this book, you will find the formulas to calculate your methionine levels for the day and a list of over 1000 foods with their methionine levels and quantities to figure out how much to eat. Do you need these calculations? It is your choice how far you want to go to reach for longevity and health.

What! You mean we have to continuously perform as a mathematician to eat on this diet?

Nope! You just eat from the top of the list.

Where To Start

Eat fruits and vegetables first and then add a small amount of legumes, seeds and nuts to round out the recipes.

Are you telling yourself, this sounds crazy!!!!

It all seems too restrictive!

Remember what we told you at the beginning of the book?

Unhealthy food is like an abusive parent, we run back to them because it is all we know. Well, now you know more! Eat fruit and vegetables, then add legumes (beans), nuts and seeds for flavor and variety. You can make the choice to never be the victim of big business again. Stop listening to the media adds and start making your own decisions!

Are, you are thinking. I can't do it?

If you want to live a longer, healthier, happier life, you can and must make these changes!

If you want to take control of the health of your DNA, your aging, your mental and psychological well being, continue to read! This book was written for you.

"Unhealthy food is like an abusive parent, we run back to them because it is all we know."

Let's make this whole thing super simple.

We will discuss proportions in greater detail later in this text. When in doubt, start with fruits and vegetables, then add small quantities of beans/ legumes, followed by an even smaller amount of nuts and seeds to maintain low dietary methionine. A food list is provided at the end of this text that lists foods with the lowest methionine at the top and greater methionine at the bottom. Make sure you look at the foods closer to the top to get an idea of which foods are the absolute lowest in methionine.

Cure For The Garden: Featuring The Methionine Restriction Protocol   Copyright 2019. DocRhi.com

How Methionine Restriction Works

Where To Start

What to drink when getting started.

Any herbal or green tea is unlimited.

- Drink only 1/2 cup or 4 oz of orange juice, vegetable juice or tomato juice per day. We pour an inch of juice into a glass of water.

- Unlimited lime or lemon water or sparkling water.

- we like to make sun tea in the summer and mix a little juice in it. we even mix a little apple juice into the stevia sweetened, almond milk cocoa we make for the kids.

- A hot cinnamon tea can be mixed with unfiltered apple juice for a winter treat.

- Naturally sparkling water and berry juice is fun and slicing cucumbers and strawberries in pure water is a beautiful way to dress up your holiday table.

We are sure your imagination can top anything that we can come up with!

What to eat when getting started.

- If it is fruit, eat it, that includes tomato, avocado, chayote, jackfruit, eggplant, tomatillo, fig, grapes, stone fruits like apple, guava, pear, cherry, berry, citrus, etc.

- Other fruit such as squash, both winter and summer, pumpkin, cucumbers, plantain, etc. use as the basis of your entrees and main dishes.

- Vegetables like brassicas and leafy greens including lettuce, cabbage, broccoli, cauliflower, kale, chard, artichoke, etc. use to make your side dishes, wrapping, noodles and dipping tools.

- Root vegetables like potatoes, jicama, carrots, turnips, taro, yam, beet, cassava, etc. can be served in slices or in recipes as flours for breads, dessert crust, or basis for dips.

How Methionine Restriction Works

Cure For The Garden: Featuring The Methionine Restriction Protocol   Copyright 2019. DocRhi.com

Where To Start

- Legumes, such as beans, peas, lentils etc. can be used as flours and dips (mixed with root and other vegetables), or can be sprouted and used for pancakes, dosas (crepes), falafel, salads or deserts. Use a pressure cooker to cook your beans when possible because pressure cooking breaks up the lignans in beans that cause flatulence.

- Nuts and seeds can be eaten as condiments, flavorings and in dips. Small amounts of nut milks can be used in recipes and as creamer in teas.

- Eating fruits and vegetables does not need to be boring or always cold and raw. It is up to you how creative you want to get!

Spices can be used liberally. Use herbs and spices as a substitute for salt. Lemon, ginger and garlic are great too!

Salt can be used according to each person's needs. The American Heart Association recommends less than 1500 mg of sodium per day. This equals about 1 teaspoon of salt for the whole day per person.

Sweeteners

- No added processed sugar is allowed!

- Simply add fruit such as dates or raisins for sweetness in your recipes.

- Stevia can be used liberally (a little at a time), agave, or maple syrup should be used sparingly.

Cure For The Garden: Featuring The Methionine Restriction Protocol   Copyright 2019. DocRhi.com

Where To Start

Fats

Avoid excessive use of oil! As a rule, add oils after cooking your food.

Do use:

- olive oil

- walnut and other nut oils

- avocado oil

These oils are the best choices for recipes and dressings. They are monounsaturated oils. This means they only have one double bond and have little danger of oxidation. Remember, oxidation can cause inflammation and aging. A little coconut oil or coconut milk can be added to recipes once you remove your food from the stove. Coconut water doesn't have a lot of fat. Remember, fats can bind to the inner walls of our blood vessels and damage them causing plaque to start forming arthrosclerosis.

Avoid frying foods. Frying foods or highly browning foods may start glycosylation, which leads to advanced aging through oxidant stress and inflammation.

How To Cook Your Food

How do I cook my food?

Baking, steaming, stewing, boiling and sautéing, as well as processing with blender, or food processor and chemically cooking with lemon, lime and fermentation are the best practices for a healthy household.

Over-browning your food can lead to a toxin called glycotoxins. Glycotoxins are a group of highly oxidizing compound known to be of significance in diabetes, heart disease and other chronic diseases. They are created with sugars and free amino groups of proteins, lipids and nucleic acid. These toxins bind to your cell surfaces or your body's proteins, and alter their structure and function causing oxidative stress and inflammation leading to disease. Consumption of a diet high in these toxins is linked to conditions such as atherosclerosis and kidney disease. **Restricting the glycotoxins you eat can prevent vascular and kidney disfunction, diabetes, can improve insulin sensitivity and accelerate wound healing.** Preventing the formation of glycotoxins can lengthen lifespan.

Remember to:

- Reduce cooking time

- Use water instead of oil in your cooking

- Cook with low temperatures

- Use lemon juice, vinegars, and other acidic ingredients including tomatoes, limes, etc. This can be as simple as using a marinade.

Eating animals and animal products, as well as grilling, broiling, searing, roasting without water, heating oils and frying, propagate and accelerate the formation of glycotoxins.

The amazing thing about eating the foods included in the Methionine Restriction Protocol is that vegetables and fruits contain very few glycotoxins even after cooking.

Reducing Glycotoxins

In review, reducing glycotoxins, reduces chronic diseases and aging. So, be sure you:

- Eat fruits and vegetables

- Lower temperatures while cooking

- Reduce cooking time

- Cook with water

- Marinade in acidic juices for 1 hour

- Use acidic ingredients such as lemon juice or vinegars in cooked foods

- Use spices and herbs, such as, ginger, cinnamon, cloves, marjoram, rosemary and tarragon

What Foods To Avoid

What not to eat on the Methionine Restriction Protocol.

The Methionine Restriction Protocol limits us to eating the fruits of the trees with seeds and the plants that have seeds.

It does **not** include:

- grasses or what we call grains,
- meat,
- eggs
- dairy, no animal products at all!
- grain oils, polyunsaturated, trans fats saturated or animal fats such as butter or lard are not used
- Avoid cooking with any saturated fats
- Avoid cooking added sugars such as honey (add small amounts after cooking)
- Avoid heating oils (add small amounts after cooking)
- Avoid processed foods, processed sugar, corn syrup, etc.
- Avoid grilling, broiling, frying and dry roasting

When we say "processed or refined" foods, we mean it is ground up, added to, preserved, colored, sweetened, fried, etc. We aren't talking about foods that are dehydrated, frozen, chopped and washed and things that don't change the structure of the plant proteins, phytochemicals and nutrients. After talking to an employee of the Department of Agriculture, we found out frozen vegetables and fruits often contain more phytonutrients than the fresh ones in the super market. This occurs because the produce is picked unripe, gassed, waxed or oiled, transported and is old by the time we purchase them.

Cure For The Garden: Featuring The Methionine Restriction Protocol   Copyright 2019. DocRhi.com

What Foods To Avoid

Why shouldn't we eat these foods?

Again, we want to reiterate, it is completely your choice what foods you eat and, if you're a parent, what your family eats. If you want to give yourself and your family the best possible probabilities for a healthy, happy long life, research demonstrates over and over eating the foods included in the Methionine Restriction Protocol is the choice to make.

Lengthy lists of phytochemicals are being packaged into nutraceutical pills for use against all types of diseases. These same phytochemicals are found in fresh, organic whole foods! And, if you are eating them regularly, they stay in your system. Fortunately for us, whole foods are packaged by nature to incur no side effects, while pharmaceuticals made from purified chemicals can cause harm. Plant chemicals contain antioxidants and chelating agents to clean our bodies of toxins including heavy metals. Eating them regularly keeps them working for us 24/7.

"Plant chemicals contain antioxidants and chelating agents to clean our bodies of toxins including heavy metals.

Another reason to choose to be free of the foods listed above is their glycotoxin content. They age us inside and out. Our skin is a reflection of the health of our organs. So, keeping our body free of glycotoxins will keep us looking and feeling younger and free of inflammation, pain and chronic diseases. Choosing to eat the foods of the Methionine Restriction Protocol keeps the body free of glycotoxins, even after cooking. Evidence demonstrates, **Methionine Restriction Protocol foods contain natures medicines for fighting environmental toxins as well as the ones we are genetically predisposed to.**

How Methionine Restriction Works

Cure For The Garden: Featuring The Methionine Restriction Protocol   Copyright 2019. DocRhi.com

An Easy Transition

Recipes for an Easy Transition

Do you remember me telling you about a fruit that tastes like blue cheese and one that chews, feels and satisfies the way meat does, without using formed protein?

Well, here are the fruits.

First the cheesy fruit is known as Noni. The problem with using Noni for the cheesy flavor is that the fresh fruit is hard to get and it ferments so easily that it doesn't ship well. You can purchase dehydrated noni fruit and use it in your dressings, as blue cheese crumbles in your salads and other dishes, and as a flavoring in things like vegan chili con queso dip.

The websites of the companies that dehydrate and sell noni have many other recipes as well!

Wringing out canned jackfruit in a cheesecloth or thin dish towel, until it is very dry will cause it to take on any flavors you cook with it and it has the consistency of pulled pork. Just add natural, no sugar added barbeque sauce and serve it as a main dish. You're family and guests will be amazed!

Breads and baked goods can be made with legumes, nuts, seeds, water chestnut and yam flours. We've included many baking recipes in the cookbook as well as recipes for vegan ice-cream, candy, and vegan grain-free mac and cheese!

How Methionine Restriction Works

Cure For The Garden: Featuring The Methionine Restriction Protocol   Copyright 2019. DocRhi.com

The First Diet And The Last You'll Ever Need

How to ensure the Methionine Restriction Protocol is the last Diet you will ever need.

Are you ready to rebel against the herd mentality of fast foods, processed meals and Oreo-like addictive foods?

Are you finished spending your money where the advertisements dictate instead of making the decision for yourself? What you put into your mouth is always your choice. Whether you eat consciously or not. is up to you. How do you become conscious of what and why you eat the things you do?

Here are a few of the Brain-Training techniques we've developed to help you transform your lifestyle.

- Start by shaking things up a little to see how changing makes you feel.

- Eat dinner for breakfast.

- Stop for a real tea break at 3 in the afternoon.

- Start keeping fruits and vegetables at your desk instead of addictive fatty, sugary, salty foods.

- Keep an individual-sized bag of seeds with you in case of a salt attack or a small baggy of nuts and raisins.

- Stop for a vegetable or fruit snack and a walk while at the job

- Keep your phone or a notebook handy and note what you eat, when and how you feel.

There is no failing! This is just a way to see how attached to foods you are, and make you more conscious of how you eat. Note how you eat as well. Do you sit stand or eat while driving? When you substitute your favorite food for another choice, does an emotion come up?

The First Diet And The Last You'll Ever Need

Write down the food you ate, when you ate it, a one word emotion and a verb for what you were doing.

Some examples might be as follows:

- cabbage wrap, breakfast, enjoyable, rushing

- banana, breakfast, dull, working

By keeping this simple 4-word food journal, you will find out your motivations and reasons for eating the way you do. We found out, we eat while working and rush every bite. We eat mostly the correct foods but never stop to enjoy them. We don't sit down to eat unless we are eating with people other than those we serve on a daily basis. We love feeling thin and light and airy but, prior to this protocol, we had achieved that goal only to have it slip away over and over. When we feel light, we feel healthier and more confident. How do your physical goals make you feel? Knowing when you mindlessly eat is the key to stopping addictive eating. Maybe, we just need to eat with more friends. My journal might say:

- chili, chives and lettuce, standing over sink, talking to husband, stuffing face

- fruit bowl, mint tea, friends, on patio.

Yes, we like the second one!

Create an image in your mind of reaching your goal, like a mental brain video to play for yourself. Take note of how do you feel? Confident and healthier? What does it look like? What are you doing? See it in vibrant detail. Don't be afraid to picture every perfect detail of what you are eating and who you are eating with. Envision your perfect life. Are you taking time to sit down at the table with friends or family in a beautiful setting with an amazing meal? Once you have the perfect mental movie, play it over and over as if rehearsing for a big show. The big show is your life and if you rehearse it enough it will be easier every day.

The First Diet And The Last You'll Ever Need

Finding a greater reason, a bigger goal is almost always the reason why people make real, lasting changes in their lives.

Once you decide that **you are the master of your own health**, getting down to the reason you want this change is really important. Without a greater conviction of some kind, when the going gets tough, we can all give in to our typical norms. Like we said before, only about 25% of people faced with chronic diseases that carry a death sentence make a lasting change.

A friend of mine helped me to understand how much comfort foods are like our parents. Jose had high cholesterol, high blood pressure, a thick waistline and was recently put on statin drugs. Even though, he was warned that he had metabolic syndrome and was heading for type 2 diabetes, he didn't change his diet and lifestyle. He was no dummy. He was the president of a collage and head of his department. But, he was still unable to make the decision to change what he ate. Why? He felt like his addictive foods comforted him. Like his mother, he felt as if ice cream and other sweets were like giving himself love. And, the more he was pushed towards healthier foods, the more angry and resistant he became. The food addiction got the better of him. He now has diabetes and is suffering the creeping effects of this silent killer. Like so many others, if he doesn't find a greater reason to chose better health, he will face Alzheimer's, possible loss of limbs and kidney failure. This is a man of great faith and belief in a Divine power. What could help him and others to make better choices? Let's find out together!

The First Diet And The Last You'll Ever Need

Finding your sacred path and following it with conviction is the path to success.

Just like Dorothy, the tin man, the lion and the scarecrow from the Wizard of Oz, The sacred path, the yellow brick road, is what they kept following. No matter what happened: a wicked witch, falling asleep, flying monkeys or a gatekeeper slamming the door to the castle, they continued towards their sacred path. Their goals were all different: to go home, get a heart, get courage or to get a brain. They shared their sacred path towards their goals, never deviating long or changing their conviction, until they finally overcome and received what they desired.

For us, our sacred path is to share the Methionine Restriction Protocol with you all again! This isn't new. It is just a reminder of what we have already been told with modern evidence of how it works. This evidence can build faith.

Build a belief in your own success.

We can start to build belief in the Methionine Restriction Protocol by including evidence from the National Institutes of Health and PubMed but that would only be a start. We can site hundreds of research articles that demonstrate that the Methionine Restriction Protocol balances metabolism, encourages fat burning, lowers blood pressure, increases insulin sensitivity, reduces pain and inflammation, retards DNA point mutations and shrinks tumors but what good would that do if you didn't belief it would help you personally?

The First Diet And The Last You'll Ever Need

Real trust begins with small victories, personal victories and appreciating each one. Once you have chosen to place your feet on the yellow brick road, **take notice of every tiny win that you or your friends and family make**.

- Did you chose fruit over cookies?

- Is your blood pressure lower?

- Did your low density lipid (LDL fat) levels drop? (Ask your doctor to measure them!)

- Is your waistline getting smaller?

- Did you prepare your lunch and walk to a park with a friend rather than go to a fast food restaurant?

- Did you clean out your cupboard and donate or throw away the sugary, fatty, processed foods?

- Did you choose to purchase only foods on The Methionine Restriction Protocol at the grocery store?

These are all successes and can be celebrated with a community on the same path. Appreciating your wins helps us believe we can reach our goals. Everyone that shares victories, no matter how small, can help others to build faith in their journey. **Share your every success! You will help someone to believe they can do it too!**

The First Diet And The Last You'll Ever Need

Community builds strength.

Together, Dorothy and the others kept each other on the yellow brick road.

Dorothy and her friends helped each other each step of the way. They gave each other courage, love, confidence and a little oiling along the way. They locked arms to hold each other up when they were down. This is what a community does for you. It helps you stay on the yellow brick road of your sacred path and make it easier to keep going when obstacles show up.

We are sure you have heard the saying, "no man is an island". This is especially true when it comes to saving your life and the lives of others. Building a team and support group is incredibly important to the success of any transition.

Like we've said before, addictive food is our comfort, our parent, what we know! **We all must realize that addictive foods will kill you slowly taking both your financial and physical wealth along the way.** Corporations formulate processed foods to cause addiction. These foods, like Oreos, are more addictive than cocaine and alcohol. And, alcoholics use the AA community to help each other transform their lives. Why not use a community to aid in our transformations?

Cure For The Garden: Featuring The Methionine Restriction Protocol   Copyright 2019. DocRhi.com

The First Diet And The Last You'll Ever Need

The proven path to kicking any bad habit is joining a group of people with like challenges.

As parents, we feel responsible for the health and happiness of our children. What if you could talk with other parents dealing with the same issues?

What if you could find another caretaker that is going through the same challenges against disease as you are?

We have a community that can help you on the path to transform your DNA and longevity. It is a community to help keep you learning and moving towards your commitment to change. The Bible tells us to gather together. It tells us this because we need others to aid each other on our sacred path, our yellow brick road towards our goal.

Our community drives us toward success!

Share:

- recipes

- substitutions

- techniques

- **tips to help transform your life, health and happiness.**

Become successful while sharing and helping others with the Methionine Restriction Protocol.

Cure For The Garden: Featuring The Methionine Restriction Protocol   Copyright 2019. DocRhi.com

Proportions

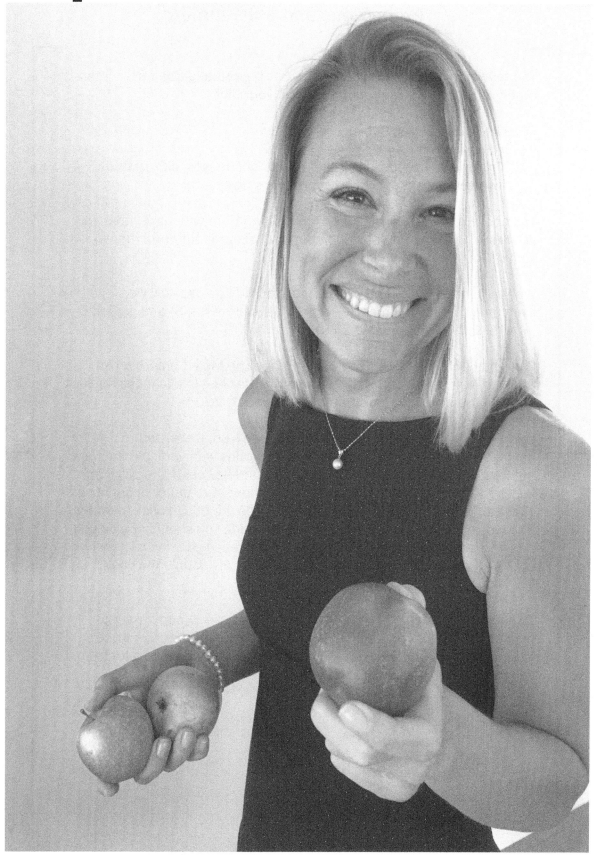

Cure For The Garden: Featuring The Methionine Restriction Protocol

Proportions and Substitutions

The following proportions can be used as a general guide for maintaining low levels of methionine in your diet.

- **65% or more - vegetables and fruit**
- **25% - legumes**
- **10% or less – seeds, nuts, nut yogurts or cheeses, oils, natural sweeteners such as agave and maple syrup**

The above portions are based on information from various doctors and studies. If you are interested in finding out more about proportions, some of our recommended resources are:

Wahls, Terry L. "Minding My Mitochondria 2nd Edition: How we overcame secondary progressive multiple sclerosis (MS) and got out of my wheelchair." Paperback. 2010

Campbell, Thomas M. II. "The China Study: The Most Comprehensive Study of Nutrition Ever Conducted and the Startling Implications for Diet, Weight Loss and Long-term Health." Hardcover. 2004

If you wish to begin incorporating more foods from trees, and to decrease gluten, you can begin to replace grains with yam, plantain and nut flour mixed with a small amount of ground flax seed and psyllium husk at a ratio of 8:1 parts flour to ground flax seed and psyllium husk. The ground flax seed and psyllium husk helps the dough stick together. Because nut flours are denser than grain flours, you should spread your dough ½ as thin when you put it in pans, decrease your oven/ grill heat by 25F degrees or to the low setting, and cook for double the cook time to make sure the dough has cooked through.

To substitute out an egg in any recipe, you can use ¼ cup flaxseed meal, 2x the recommended baking soda with 1 tablespoon of white vinegar. To achieve fluffiness you can whisk agua faba, the water from a can of garbanzo beans until it holds peaks like meringue (About 5 minutes on high) and add it to the flax seed meal, baking soda, and vinegar.

Cure For The Garden: Featuring The Methionine Restriction Protocol

Easy Example Breakfasts

Meal Plans

Breakfast is definitely our favorite meal! Be sure to check out hot cakes, root hash, and sunflower hot cereal from the breakfast and baked goods section of the cookbook. When we take the time to make those meals we usually repurpose the leftovers (i.e. Root hash cabbage wraps with beans and guacamole for dinner). When you make baked goods, freeze them and take them out the night before to defrost for breakfast!
All recipes for meal plans can be found in the recipe section of The Methionine Restriction Protocol text.

Breakfast 1:

A hearty fresh fruit salad with apples, pears, berries, cherries, grapes, oranges, kiwi, and ripe banana. Squeeze in the juice of a lemon or orange, and add cinnamon, ginger, and nutmeg to taste. Top with shredded coconut.

1 small grain-free vegan muffin

Hot tea creamed with homemade tahini milk

Breakfast 2:

1/2 a cantaloupe or honeydew melon (deseeded)
*Note that melon and squash seeds can be saved in the refrigerator or dried out for longer storage and eaten 5-10 seeds at a time for constipation.

1/2 cup coconut yogurt inside of your melon

Top with raisins or dried cherries

1 slice of grain-free vegan toast

Hot tea creamed with homemade tahini or sunflower seed milk

Breakfast 3:

1 large baked/boiled/ or steamed yam topped with sea salt and 1/2 teaspoon raw coconut oil

1 orange or grapefruit

1 cup of homemade tahini or sunflower seed milk steamer

Cure For The Garden: Featuring The Methionine Restriction Protocol   Copyright 2019. DocRhi.com

Easy Example Lunches and Dinners

Meal 1:

Red potatoes and greens steamed with salt, pepper and paprika

Apple sliced with nut/ seed butter and cinnamon

Stevia sweetened lemon or limeade

Meal 2:

Lentil falafel with hummus, carrots, celery, jicama, cauliflower, and lettuce spears
*Note, if you have a tendency towards abdominal pain or bloating you should dry heat your fresh veggies for 2 minutes and add digestive spices such as cumin and coriander instead of eating raw. This will increase the digestibility of your food.

Fennel tea with nut or seed milk, cinnamon, and nutmeg (You can literally just make this tea from your kitchen spices!)

Meal 3:

Stir-sautéed vegetables with avocados, arugula, sunflower or sesame seeds

Sliced Pear with chocolate raspberry drizzle

Mint tea sweetened with stevia leaves

Easy Example Snacks

Aztec Fudge

Berry Cherry Ice Cream

Dates with Vegan Cream Cheese (purchase at health food store)

Tapioca Pudding

Hot Cocoa

Grain-free Granola

Grain-free Cereal

Kale Chips

When in doubt, have an apple! And, make sure you eat before you get to the point of starving! Keeping snacks around will help you to make healthy choices! Always add as much produce as possible to nuts and seeds when you are snacking in order to keep methionine levels low.

Cure For The Garden: Featuring The Methionine Restriction Protocol   Copyright 2019. DocRhi.com

Grocery List

Vegetables
Dried chilies (enchilada sauce)
Serrano chilies
Jalapenos
Pasillas chilies
Green red bell peppers
Tomatillos
Chives
Tomatoes
Eggplant
Zucchini
Yellow squash
Spaghetti squash
Acorn squash
Cabbage
Cilantro
Parsley
Carrots
Chard
Romaine lettuce
Avocado
Cucumber
Sauerkraut
Cornichons (little French pickles)
Broccoli
Cauliflower
Crushed tomatoes
Tomato paste
Grape leaves
Sliced black olives
Onions, red and brown
Kale
Okra
Yam (Iyan) flour
Plantain flour
Hearts of palm
Dried shiitake mushrooms
Green jackfruit
Water chestnut (Singoda) flour
Cheote (Mexican) squash

Fruit (Local and in season)
Lemons
Limes
Berries (frozen and fresh)
Pineapple
Raisins
Pears
Dates (pitted if possible)
Kiwis
Mangos
Cherries
Apples
Cherries
Melons

Spices & Add-ons
Ginger
Sea salt
Cumin
Coriander
Cayenne
Fennel
Dill
Tamari sauce
Sugarless hot/ jalapeño sauce
White pepper
Horseradish
Paprika
Black pepper corns
Cardamom
Cinnamon sticks and ground
Cloves whole and ground
Nutmeg
Wasabi
Turmeric
Thyme
Mint
Oregano
Curry powder
Coconut aminos

Cure For The Garden: Featuring The Methionine Restriction Protocol   Copyright 2019. DocRhi.com

Grocery List

Basil, fresh
Cilantro, fresh
Aluminum-free baking powder & soda
Pectin (No sugar needed type)
Coconut aminos
Garlic powder and crushed or fresh
Balsamic vinegar
Apple cider vinegar
White vinegar
Mustard (without sugar)

Legumes
Mung (or moong)
Lentils
Organic raw cacao bars and baking cocoa
Organic non-GMO miso
Organic non-GMO extra firm and soft tofu
Mung/ Edamame/ Lentil (Udad) noodles & flours
Chickpea (Besan) flour
Black/ Kidney/ Pinto/ White beans
Fat free, vegetarian refried beans
Canned garbanzo beans

Vegan dairy
Vegan Cheese
Vegan Cream Cheese
Coconut Yogurt
Nutritional Yeast

Nuts and seeds
Almond flour
Psyllium husk (Look in the vitamin section)
Almond butter
Peanut butter
Flaxseed Meal
Tahini paste

Slivered almonds
Sunflower seeds
Cashews
Sesame seeds
Walnuts
Pecans
Chia seeds
Unsweetened Coconut Shreds
Unsweetened Cocoa Powder

Oils
Extra virgin olive oil
Coconut oil
Sesame oil
Almond oil

Sweeteners
Ground stevia leaf (not anything with added milk, mannose or dextrose!)
Organic raw agave
All fruit spread
Maple Syrup

Beverages
Hemp, Coconut or Almond milk
Tea (green, rooibos, or herbal)/ Swiss water acid-free decaffeinated coffee
Natural sparkling water

Prepared Snacks (Optional)
Lara bars (without sugar, dates ok)
Unsweetened dried fruit
Coconut Bliss / "Nada Moo" ice-cream

Cure For The Garden: Featuring The Methionine Restriction Protocol

Intro

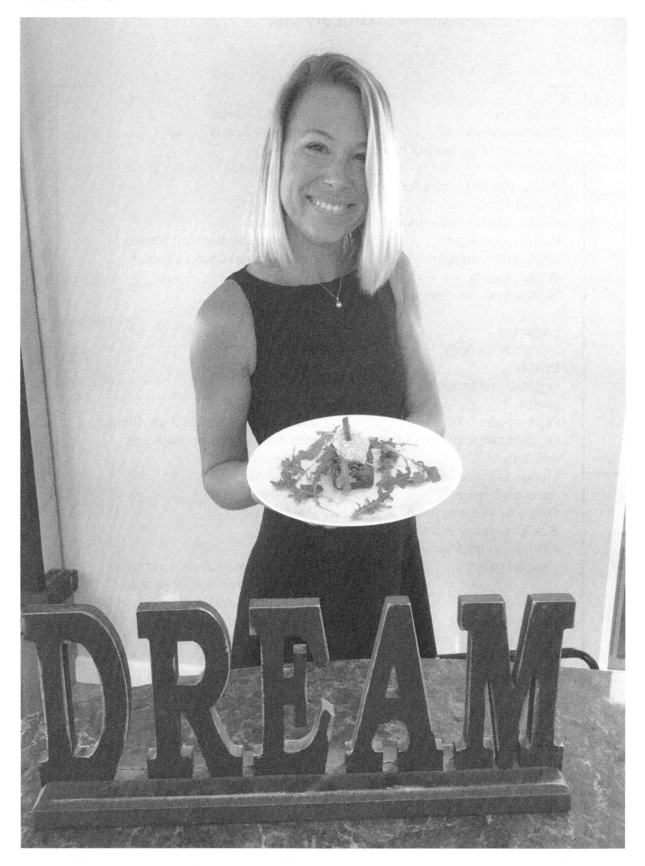

Cure For The Garden: Featuring The Methionine Restriction Protocol

What To Eat When You Don't Feel Like Cooking

Many times, when you get home late, are running to a party or need an after school snack you simply don't have a lot of prep-time. This is a list of simple foods you can make or tell others about who want to learn how to get started with eating a vegan, grain-free diet.

- Hummus and fresh vegetables
- Salsa and jicama slices
- Vegan refried beans mixed with tomatoes, onions, peppers, cilantro, and celery sticks (Vegan cheese or coconut yogurt optional)
- Steamed broccoli with mushrooms, and sea salt
- Roasted cauliflower and tahini sauce
- Grilled fresh vegetables with tamari and balsamic vinegar or a citrus marinade
- Baked potatoes with baked garlic cloves and sea salt or broccoli
- Any kind of roasted vegetables with roasted garlic, onions and sea salt
- Sautéed mixed vegetables with a mild salsa and serve over crumbled cauliflower or black beans
- Baked apples with cinnamon and nutmeg (raisins if you like)
- Artichokes with lemon and sea salt
- Of course, salads and soups of fruits, vegetables and lentils are welcome too. Having both cooked and raw foods is necessary to help to satisfy hunger and gives you more available nutrients. My favorite quick salad is chopped tomato, cucumber and avocado mixed with lemon juice and sea salt, and served with romaine lettuce spears. Simple and delicious.
- An easy dressing for any salad is a smashed avocado, lemon juice and sea salt. Mix and toss with the salad.
- You can also purchase premade olive tapenade, pesto, hummus, baba ghanoush, and other salads and dips but make sure you read the ingredients for cane and hidden sugars (anything ending in –ose other than fruit sugar fructose) and dairy products.
- Precook lentils or lentil soup and freeze in individual servings
- Baked yam with oranges and cinnamon

Cure For The Garden: Featuring The Methionine Restriction Protocol   Copyright 2019. DocRhi.com

Save Money By Storing Food Properly

The first thing you can do to help you keep your produce longer is to hand select it. Shop local and buy your produce in different stages of ripeness. Check your produce daily for softness, ripeness and pocked ones and remove them to eat first.

Did you know that root vegetables will keep for months in cool sand. You can purchase clean sand at toys are us and pour it into plastic keepers. Then just bury carrots, beets, turnips, potatoes etc. in the sand. They like to be cool, dry and dark. If you live in a humid and warm area be aware that your produce may ripen faster. Try to keep them dry and cool.

To keep onions fresh, take old panty hose and slide one in, tie a knot and then add the next one. Hang them up and when ready, cut the bottom knot to free the bottom one. Make sure your knots are tight though! Garlic likes to be kept by themselves in a cool, dry and dark place too! in a bottom drawer or cupboard. Green onions or scallions can be kept on a window sill in a cup of water like a flower. They will continue to grow if you trim the green from the top as needed and leave the white in the water.

Use large, heavy mason jars to store food in the refrigerator. Cut lettuce and place into the jar with a dry paper towel in the refrigerator. They like cool and moist.

Store apples in the bottom drawer away from other vegetables and fruits. Be sure to separate the bruised apples, "One bad apple can spoil the whole bunch girl". Slice and dehydrate the bruised ones, or throw ripe fresh fruits and vegetables into boiling water, drain and freeze to store for long periods. We do this with apples and peaches and have them for desserts and smoothies all year.

Wrap the stems of your bananas with plastic wrap to contain the ethylene gas from spreading and ripening other fruit to fast. Also store them separately too. Peel your ripe bananas and store in the freezer. They are easier to get out if you freeze them first on a tray separately and then put them all together.

Rinse berries and cucumbers in 1 part vinegar and 5 parts water, dry and store in paper cover bowls in refrigerator.

Cure For The Garden: Featuring The Methionine Restriction Protocol   Copyright 2019. DocRhi.com

Save Money By Storing Food Properly

You can chop and freeze fresh herbs or you can hang them in a well ventilated area to dry. You can even put them into your dehydrator! Then put into jars with your dried spices. Ginger can be ground or graded and froze in ice trays inside freezer bags and kept for months.

Use heavy mason jars like the brand name Ball to freeze in. Remember to leave at least an inch or two empty because things expand and contract when freezing and thawing. Store the jars upside down to create a airtight seal just remember to make sure to tighten the lid first. Keep your refrigerator between 35-38 degrees F for best results.
You can purchase ethylene gas absorbers to collect the gases ripe fruit put off. This helps stop the unripe fruit from ripening to fast. On the other hand, if you want a fruit to ripen, put it with a ripe fruit to help it along.

Place your nuts and seeds into mason jars and keep them in the refrigerator if them are already shelled. This will keep them from molding or going rancid. In their shells, nuts can stay in a cool dry place for a long time. Buy them in the shell and that way you will eat less. we also keep my flours in mason jars!

Store citrus fruit by laying in one layer and look for the ripest, softest ones first. If you see rot, cut it off and use it now. Citrus can be stored in the refrigerator for long periods. Racks in your frig is a good idea.
Use your mangos when their skins are getting wrinkled. Freeze or dehydrate them. Papayas don't ripen after they are picked so buy them ripe and eat them, freeze or dehydrate right away. Check your avocados daily and place the soft ones into the refrigerator and use asap. Squashes, pumpkins, sweet potatoes can be placed in a cool dry place for a long period.

Don't store tomatoes in the refrigerator but pick out the ripe one right away and use.

Juice your watermelons for a great drink and good firm ones will last a long time. Young coconuts still in the husks will store a long time but check for leaking.

Grow your greens and pick only the leaves off as you need them.

Compost your leftovers and rotten produce.

Cure For The Garden: Featuring The Methionine Restriction Protocol   Copyright 2019. DocRhi.com

The Art of Spicing

These spice ideas are just an easy way of spicing things to taste like a certain ethnic food. These are very simple ideas, and are certainly not the only way to season for the different cultural foods. we always use fresh spices when we can. When using the recipes, if you want onions, use the ones suggested. The spices listed first are the most important, but all are really good. Just use the rules and have fun.

Herbs just as foods, lose their phytonutrients over time. So **if you have herbs in your cupboard that are older than 1 year, throw them out!!!**

- Mexican Food: cumin, oregano, chili powder (easy on this one), black pepper, sea salt, lemon or lime juice, garlic, onion and fresh cilantro, optional deseeded green chilies.

- Italian Food: basil, oregano, fennel seed, thyme, rosemary, parsley, garlic, onion, sea salt, a dash of stevia if using tomato sauce/paste, etc.

"We always use fresh spices when we can.."

- Mediterranean Food: coriander, cumin, sumac, sesame seeds, red chilies, pepper, garlic, lemon juice, fresh parsley, red onions, sea salt. Use extra virgin olive oil and paprika on top.

- Asian Food: cilantro, basil (Holy basil if you can get it), lemon grass or lemon juice, white pepper, fresh ginger, garlic, red chilies flakes, tamari sauce, miso, green onions, kaffir lime leaves.

- Indian/ Pakistani Food: turmeric, cumin, coriander, deseeded green peppers, white onion, cinnamon stick, garlic, black mustard seed, lemon juice, sea salt, fresh cilantro, fennel seeds, olive oil, green mango or tamarind.

Cure For The Garden: Featuring The Methionine Restriction Protocol   Copyright 2019. DocRhi.com

From Scratch

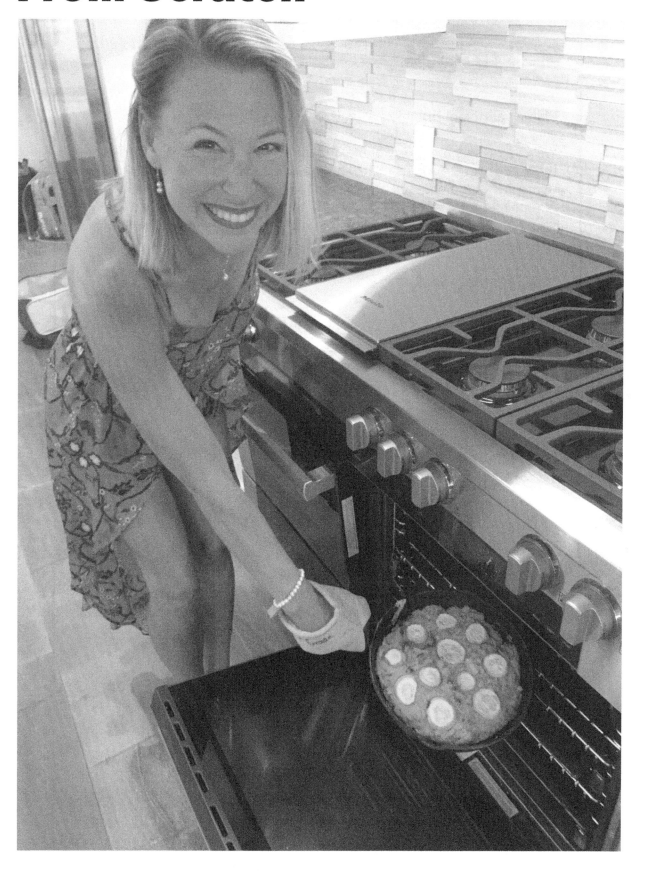

Cure For The Garden: Featuring The Methionine Restriction Protocol   Copyright 2019. DocRhi.com

Un-processing Your Food

From Scratch

Make It at Home! Nut milks, yogurt, chips, and more...

We love to have the luxury of making things for ourselves. You can feel the energy of the food as it lifts your mood as soon as you eat homemade, unprocessed, un-shelfed foods. As shelf time (the amount of time food sits on a shelf) increases, the phytonutrients or plant nutrients decrease, so if you are low on energy or healing, try boosting your energy by un-processing your food!

Seed and Nut Milk

- 4 or 5 cups water
- 1/2 cup seeds or nuts
- Vanilla extract (optional)
- Agave or stevia (optional)

Put all ingredients in a pan; bring water to a full boil. Fill blender halfway with ingredients, cover with lid and towel, and blend together on low, then high. Strain through a cheesecloth. Repeat until all liquid has been blended. If too thick, add more boiling water. Refrigerate. **For a quicker milk you can just blend 2 tablespoons tahini or nut butter in a high speed blender with 1 1/2 cups milk and vanilla and stevia optionally.**

"If you are low on energy or healing, try boosting your energy by un-processing your food.."

Cure For The Garden: Featuring The Methionine Restriction Protocol   Copyright 2019. DocRhi.com

Un-processing Your Food

From Scratch

If you are allergic to nuts, you can substitute tahini (sesame seed paste) or sunflower seed butter.

Nut Creamer or Steamer

Put all ingredients in a single serving cup for the blender and mix until completely smooth.

Pour into tea or coffee instead of sugary, milky, store-bought, expensive creamers!

If you want to make a steamer, increase the banana to 1/2 and steam for a non-caffeinated, warm and wonderful treat that is great for kids. Pour leftovers into ice tray and freeze for use in ice cream recipes or more creamer for later.

- 2 Tablespoons organic almond butter (unsweetened)
- 1 cup of water
- 1/4 of a ripe banana
- Nutmeg, cinnamon, and stevia to taste

"A non-caffeinated, warm and wonderful treat that is great for kids!"

Cure For The Garden: Featuring The Methionine Restriction Protocol   Copyright 2019. DocRhi.com

Un-processing Your Food

Nut, Seed, or Chickpea Cheese

We find that having a cheese substitute is one of the most important necessities to changing your diet. You can use any nut, seed, or garbanzo bean flour and probably other bean flours as well. You can season sweet cheese spreads or make savory cheese logs like the one we like! Have fun with your spices and ingredients and don't be afraid to experiment.

Soak your nuts/seeds overnight, rinse and drain. Combine kombucha and nuts or seeds in a high-speed blender individual cup and blend until creamy. Place into a bowl and cover with a plate to leave out for 36 hours. Blend with spices and move into wax paper and roll it into a log. Top with desired nuts or seeds. Twist both sides of the wax paper and place into refrigerator for 4-6 days. Enjoy within 1 week.

- 1 cup nuts or seeds (soaked overnight and drained) or use bean flour with 1 tablespoon tahini

- 3 tablespoons any kombucha

- 1 teaspoon salt

- Spices of choice (Try garlic and onion chives, bagel spices, herbs de Provence, nutritional yeast, peppercorns, jalapeño, or try a sweet spread with stevia, agave and dried unsweetened cherries)

- Top with almond slivers/ sesame seeds (optional)

If you use bean flour instead of nuts you need to slowly whisk 3/4-1 cup water with bean flour and tahini and bring to a boil. Remove from heat and mix with kombucha and proceed as above.

If you love pepper jack like we do, try seasoning with red pepper flakes, serrano chilis, nutritional yeast, lemon juice, and cumin.

Cure For The Garden: Featuring The Methionine Restriction Protocol   Copyright 2019. DocRhi.com

Make Your Food Make More Food

Sprouting

One of the nice things about using sprouted legumes, such as lentils, is that it increases all proteins except methionine! Also, once you sprout legumes, they don't really need to be cooked. We like to dehydrate some of our recipes and sprouting your legumes before you cook with them will help them to stick together. Another great reason to sprout is that it extends your food exponentially and that saves you money!

Sprouts

Place 1/4 cup of lentils into a large sprouting jar. Fill the jar 3/4 with water (preferably chlorine-free water) and let stand overnight. Pour out the water in the morning and rinse the lentils morning and night until they have sprouted. Sprouting timing depends on the temperature the lentils are sitting in. They like it about 70 F. Drain and let stand before using to get rid of the excess water and use in recipes.

- 1 large sprouting jar or a large jar with netting and a rubber band to let them breathe and drain easily.

- 1/2 cup lentils or other legume such as mung

- water (optional chlorine-free)

"Sprouting extends your food exponentially and that saves you money.!.."

Cure For The Garden: Featuring The Methionine Restriction Protocol   Copyright 2019. DocRhi.com

Using A Dehydrator

Dehydration

We absolutely love our dehydrator. Yes, you can dehydrate fruit, yes you can make your own chips and cracker, but you can also use it for small pancakes, falafels, and veggie-patties. Dehydrating helps to maintain the enzymes in the food, which helps you to break them down more easily!

General Instructions for Drying Fruit

Use any kind of fruit. Wash, slice thinly and uniformly. Place on dehydrator screen. Change positions of shelves once a day so that they dehydrate evenly. When fruit reaches leather-hard, remove from shelves and enjoy.

- 1 kale bunch
- 1 tablespoons tamari or coconut aminos
- 1 tablespoon balsamic vinegar
- 1/2 teaspoon white pepper

Kale chips

Wash a bunch of kale, then shake it and let it dry. De-vein the leaves from the center vein. In a plastic bag mix 1 tablespoon each of tamari sauce and balsamic vinegar with ½ teaspoon each of white pepper and curry powder. Or, try almond butter, nutritional yeast and salt. Place the leaves in bags and shake to mix altogether. Make sure there are no holes in the bag. Place in dehydrator or low oven at 100F degrees until crispy. They must be eaten right away or they will get soft.

"Dehydrating helps to maintain the enzymes in the food.."

Cure For The Garden: Featuring The Methionine Restriction Protocol   Copyright 2019. DocRhi.com

Using A Dehydrator

Savory Sprouted Lentil Juice-Shred Crackers

Pulse leftover juicing shreds in a food processor until well shredded. Place lentils, shreds, raisins and seasonings into food processor and pulse, stirring as necessary. Roll into balls and flatten dough as thin as possible. Place each onto dehydrator trays and dry until crunchy.

- 1 cup sprouted lentils
- 1 cup vegetable and fruit juicing shreds
- 1/4 cup raisins
- 1 tablespoon tamari
- 1 tablespoon balsamic vinegar
- 1 tablespoon minced garlic
- 1 teaspoon sea salt
- 1 teaspoon white pepper or chili flakes

Cure For The Garden: Featuring The Methionine Restriction Protocol   Copyright 2019. DocRhi.com

Breakfast

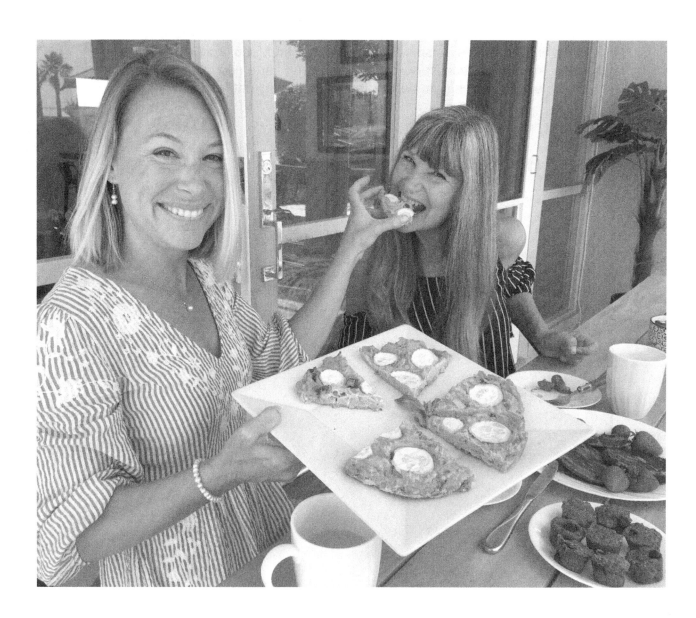

Truly A Breakfast of Champions

Breakfast

According to some of the largest nutrition studies ever conducted, one should never eat too much raw or cold food. This rule especially applies to breakfast when the body is setting up its metabolism for the day. So eat something warm in the morning & sit down to you're your body digest and de-stress. Often times we will make our batter for the week as a simple crepe batter. We make crepes on the weekend. The next day, we will use some of the leftover batter that we refrigerated and add some walnuts or sunflower seeds, raisins, and cinnamon and stick it in an oiled muffin pan. Because it is now thicker, it cooks nicely in the muffin pans. Bake at 300F degrees, for about 20-25 minutes, or until a knife stuck in one of the muffins is not wet with batter. The day after that we will use more of the leftovers and add some fruit that is getting old, with a few heaping tablespoons of baking cocoa and a sweetener like maple syrup. This time we spread it thinly in an oiled bread pan and bake about 35 minutes, at 300F. Turn the oven off and let the bread cool for an hour. Your friends will think you slaved all day to bake!

- 2 cups of almond, plantain, moong bean or yam flour
- 1 tablespoon psyllium husk
- 1 tablespoon ground flax seed
- 1 can of water from garbanzo beans (This is called agua faba)
- 1 teaspoon salt
- 2 cups of nut milk
- 1 tablespoon organic agave

Sweet or Savory Crepes

Whisk garbanzo water on high for 9 minutes or until it holds peaks. Add all other ingredients. If too thick, add more liquid. Use a non-stick skillet or coat a skillet with just enough olive or grapeseed oil to line the pan using a cloth napkin. Pre-heat the skillet with oil. Use a ladle to pour one crepe at a time into the pan. Cook on medium heat until bubbles pop on the top and edges turn slightly golden. Then turn over and do the same. Remove from pan and fill with whatever filling you wish. Repeat until all the batter has been used, or store the batter in the refrigerator for up to four days. For savory vegetable lunch or dinner crepes, eliminate agave.

Cure For The Garden: Featuring The Methionine Restriction Protocol   Copyright 2019. DocRhi.com

Truly A Breakfast of Champions

Granola Breakfast Cookies (With Leftover Crepe Batter)

Combine all ingredients in a mixing bowl. Spoon 1 tablespoon sized cookies onto a non-stick cookie sheet. Bake at 300F for 30 minutes, turn oven off and allow to stay in hot oven for 30 more minutes.

- 1 cup crepe batter (See previous recipe)
- 1 diced apple
- 1 chopped banana
- 1/8 cup each raisins, chopped and dried unsweetened cherries, goji berries, raw sunflower seeds, and unsweetened coconut shreds
- 1/2 teaspoon nutmeg, pumpkin pie spice, salt
- 1 teaspoon dry or 6 liquid drops of stevia to taste
- 1/4 cup chopped or sliced nuts (optional)

Cure For The Garden: Featuring The Methionine Restriction Protocol

Truly A Breakfast of Champions

Blintz Filling for Crepes

In a high speed blender, pulse raisins and dates until gummy then add berries, tofu, lemon juice and pulse again several times until a creamy or ricotta texture is achieved depending upon the tofu hardness you used. We love the traditional extra firm tofu for that traditional ricotta texture but some people prefer more of a creamy smooth texture which is achieved with creamy tofu.

- 1 package of tofu (soft for creamy filling or extra firm for traditional ricotta texture)
- 1 tablespoon organic agave
- 1 cup frozen raspberry's or other berry
- 1 cup mixed raisins and pitted dates
- Stevia to taste
- Juice of 1/4 lemon

Breakfast

Truly A Breakfast of Champions

Good Morning Hot Cereal

This is one of our favorite breakfasts and we will often make extra for the whole week. Pulse sunflower seeds in a high speed blender individual cup until coarsely chopped. Mix dates, sunflower seeds, dried fruit, nuts/ seeds and spices and leave in a mason jar until the night before you are ready to use. The night before you want to have your hot cereal for breakfast, take the amount you would like out of the jar and soak overnight by covering it completely with water. In the morning heat until warm. Add apple, banana and seed/nut milk as needed.

- 1 cup shelled sunflower seeds
- 6 pitted dates, chopped fine
- 1/4 cup flax seed meal
- 1 diced apple
- 1 chopped banana
- 1/4 cup each raisins, chopped and dried unsweetened cherries, goji berries, and unsweetened coconut shreds
- 1/2 teaspoon cinnamon and salt
- 1-2 teaspoons dry or 6 liquid drops of stevia to taste
- 1/8 cup chopped dried, unsweetened mango (optional)

Serves 3-4.

You may also serve over plain coconut milk yogurt and berries or berry all fruit. For a sweet treat you can drench muesli in the homemade steamer (See from Scratch section).

Truly A Breakfast of Champions

Apple Pan Betty with Blueberry Sorbet

This is like an apple pie with blueberry ice cream, except it is so good for you that you can eat it for breakfast!

On medium-low heat, dry roast chestnut flour for about 10 minutes or until it turns golden. In a separate bowl, whisk agua faba for about 9 minutes on high or until it holds peaks like merengue. Add all other dry ingredients to chestnut flour. In a separate bowl combine all wet ingredients except agua faba and drench diced apples in the wet mixture. Add the apple mixture to the dry and fold in agua faba. Place in oiled and floured cast iron skillet and bake for 45 minutes to 1 hour at 300F.

Serves 5-6. Top with berry sorbet!

- 1 1/2 cup roasted chestnut flour
- 1 tablespoon each milled flax and psyllium husk
- 1 can agua faba (whisked water from a can of garbanzo beans)
- 6 diced apples
- 1/3 cup raisins
- 1/3 cup maple syrup
- 2 teaspoons cinnamon
- 1 teaspoon pumpkin pie spice
- 12 drops stevia
- 2 tablespoons white vinegar
- 1/4 cup sparkling water

Berry Sorbet

Place 1/8 cup nut milk in the bottom of a food processor with stevia and agave to taste then (We use 1 tablespoon agave and 10 drops of liquid stevia) add 1 cup blueberries or other berry and process on high for a couple of minutes or until an ice cream consistency. You may optionally add 1 banana and reduce the agave and stevia.

Cure For The Garden: Featuring The Methionine Restriction Protocol — Copyright 2019. DocRhi.com

Truly A Breakfast of Champions

Hot Muesli and Cold Cereal

In one large pan, combine flax and psyllium, stir and heat on medium heat. add other ingredients and heat until golden.

If you are not up for cooking, you can skip the heating and simply mix up all of the ingredients in a bowl and add homemade nut milk but it is better for digestion to heat for at least 2 minutes.

- 2 tablespoons tahini
- 1/2 cup sliced almonds, chopped walnuts or other nut
- 1/2 cup raisins, or other dried fruit
- 1/4 cup flax seed
- 1/8 cup psyllium husk
- 1/4 cup hulled sunflower seeds
- 1/4 cup unsweetened coconut (optional)
- 1 teaspoon cinnamon
- 1/2 teaspoon nutmeg
- Sea salt to taste

Cure For The Garden: Featuring The Methionine Restriction Protocol   Copyright 2019. DocRhi.com

Truly A Breakfast of Champions

Root Hash

Preheat oven to 425F and preheat an oven-safe skillet on the stovetop on medium heat. Add 2 tablespoons of water to the preheated skillet, then add onions. Cook until onions are transparent. Add garlic and spices and stir thoroughly. Add all other ingredients and stir to coat all vegetables. Add 2 tablespoons of water to bottom of pan. Place lid on pan and roast for 30-35 minutes, then remove lid and cook 10-15 minutes more or until golden on top and the vegetable are easy to pierce with a fork. Top with paprika, marinated onions, Pico de Gallo or salsa and serve for breakfast, lunch or dinner.

- 1 beet root
- 3 carrots
- 1 red onion
- 4 potatoes
- 1 turnip root
- 1 heaping tablespoon garlic
- 1 1/2 teaspoons sea salt
- 1 teaspoon black pepper
- 1/4 teaspoon chili flakes
- 1 teaspoon parsley flakes
- 1 teaspoon rosemary
- 1 teaspoon thyme
- paprika
- 4 tablespoons water
- 1 teaspoon sage (optional)

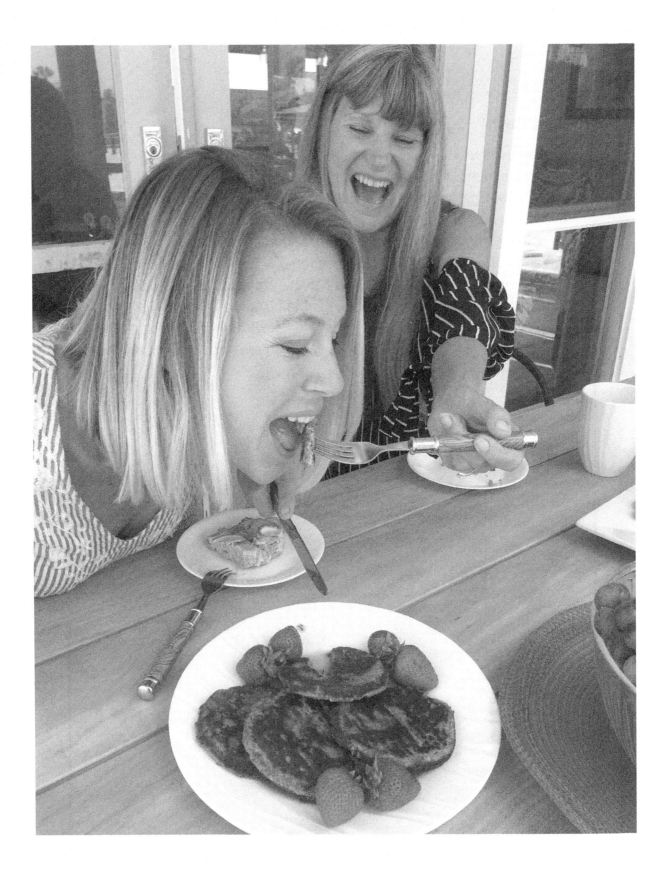

Cure For The Garden: Featuring The Methionine Restriction Protocol

Truly A Breakfast of Champions

Breakfast

The Ultimate Hot Cakes

These are our favorite breakfast for dinner item. They can be topped with almost anything or are good all by themselves! Make them on the weekend and refrigerate for a great weekday snack!

- 2 cups of almond, plantain, chickpea or yam flour
- 1 tablespoon psyllium husk
- 1 tablespoon ground flax seed
- 1 can of water from garbanzo beans (agua faba)
- 2 beaten or mashed ripe bananas
- 1 tablespoon white vinegar
- 1 tablespoon of raw agave
- 2 teaspoons dried ground stevia or 6 drops, to taste
- 1 teaspoon baking powder
- 1 teaspoon baking soda
- 1/2 teaspoon cinnamon and salt
- 1/4 teaspoon cloves and nutmeg
- 1/8 teaspoon dried ginger
- 1/2 - 1 cup cold sparkling water (depending upon the flour used)

Drain water from 1 can of plain organic garbanzo beans into a mixing bowl. Using electric mixer, mix starting at low and moving to high to not make a mess. Beat on highest level or meringue setting , 9 minutes, or until stiff and holds peaks.

In another bowl combine all dry ingredients and mix well. Add all wet ingredients then fold in agua faba. If consistency is too thick to pour into hot cakes, add more sparkling water.

Grain-free flours tend to cook more slowly so cook in a non-stick skillet on <u>low heat</u>. They are worth waiting for!

Cure For The Garden: Featuring The Methionine Restriction Protocol   Copyright 2019. DocRhi.com

The Secret To Going Vegan Is In The Special Sauce!

Sauces

Guacamole

Mix all together in a bowl or, if you don't want to hand chop your ingredients, you can pulse all ingredients except the avocados in a food processor then add avocado a pulse quickly.

Optionally, for Cabbage Salad, add the juice of one lemon and head of 1 green cabbage, chopped, to the above. Refrigerate overnight. Serve chilled.

- 1 small purple onion chopped finely
- 4 large tomatoes chopped
- 4 large ripe avocados, smashed
- 1/2 bunch cilantro, finely chopped
- 5 cloves crushed garlic
- 2 limes, juiced
- 1/8 cup fresh oregano
- 1 teaspoon cumin
- 1 teaspoon sea salt
- 1/2 teaspoon black pepper
- 1 deseeded, minced jalapeño

Hint For Making The Jump To Vegan***

Choose your favorite foods and find ways to substitute one thing at a time. Try starting with the Bean Burgers and using the burger patties broken up as a ground meat substitute. Or, try topping with vegan cheese or nutritional yeast. Remember that you still want that coziness factor so select creamy toppings such as guacamole or vegan alfredo.

Also reinforce why you are making these changes each morning with an affirmation "I am as healthy and as beautiful as what I put in my body!"

Optional: Save half the guacamole to use on fajitas the next day.

Cure For The Garden: Featuring The Methionine Restriction Protocol   Copyright 2019. DocRhi.com

The Secret To Going Vegan Is In The Special Sauce!

Sauces

Pico De Gallo

In a bowl, mix ingredients thoroughly with lemon juice and let sit for 1 hour before serving.

This recipe can be mixed with avocados for a quick guacamole or added to the Vegan Mayonnaise for a creamy dip!

If you are a fan of fresh mango, substitute it for the tomatoes and use it to top vegan burger lettuce wraps for a tropical treat!

- 3 tomatoes, diced
- 1 small onion, diced
- 1/8 cup chopped cilantro or more to taste
- 1 lemon juiced
- 1 deseeded jalapeno pepper, diced
- 2 sweet peppers, diced
- 1 teaspoon sea salt
- 1/2 cucumber diced (optional)
- A pinch of red chili flakes and boiled, diced tomatillos (optional)

The Secret To Going Vegan Is In The Special Sauce!

Sauces

Roasted Garlic Salsa

Preheat oven to 425 F. Place all ingredients except spices, lime and cilantro into roasting pan, cover and bake 25 minutes. Remove lid and bake 15 more minutes. Deseed peppers and chilies. Place onions, green onions, peppers and chilies into food processor and pulse until well chopped. Add the rest of the roasted ingredients, spices and cilantro and pulse. Add lime juice and pulse. Chill and serve.

Serve with lightly salted celery, carrot sticks, jicama, or dehydrated plantain chips or sweet potato chips as a substitute for tortilla chips.

- 3 tomatoes

- 3 tomatillos

- 1 brown onion

- 2 green onions

- 1 whole garlic bulb

- 1 jalapenos more if you like spicy hot

- 2 Anaheim chilies

- 1 teaspoon sea salt

- 1 teaspoon cumin

- 1 teaspoon oregano

- 1/2 cayenne

- 1/8 cup cilantro

- juice of 2 limes

Cure For The Garden: Featuring The Methionine Restriction Protocol   Copyright 2019. DocRhi.com

The Secret To Going Vegan Is In The Special Sauce!

Sauces

Enchilada Sauce

Place all ingredients into a blender. Be sure to finely filter out any remaining chili seeds so that your enchilada sauce isn't too hot. Let sit several minutes, and then blend on high until blender gets hot. Pour into a bowl or pitcher. Serves 8.

Use to dip or top steamed veggies, with banana or yam chips, or with grain-free tortillas and vegan cheese.

Or, pour over chard, fresh vegetables, such as broccoli, potatoes, carrots, zucchini and beans and bake for in the oven for 25 minutes at 325F for vegan enchiladas! We like to top tofu, spinach, mushrooms and black olives with this sauce and bake, covered for 15 minutes at 350F. Top with nutritional yeast.

- 1 package dried chili pasilla, de-seeded and de-stemmed

- 2 packages California chili pods, de-seeded and de-stemmed

- 3 cups boiling water

- 1 can organic tomatoes

- Sea salt to taste

- 3 garlic cloves, crushed

- 1 tablespoon each oregano and cumin

Cure For The Garden: Featuring The Methionine Restriction Protocol   Copyright 2019. DocRhi.com

The Secret To Going Vegan Is In The Special Sauce!

Sauces

Tzatziki Cucumber Dip

- 2 cups coconut or cashew yogurt
- 1/2 cup cucumbers, finely chopped and dried on a towel
- 1/8 cup red onion chopped very fine
- 1 tablespoon balsamic vinegar
- 1 tablespoon fresh chopped dill
- 4 fresh garlic cloves, crushed
- Sea salt to taste

Mix ingredients by hand and chill in the refrigerator so the flavors blend for 1 hour. Serve with fresh chopped veggies, as a salad dressing, or on sprouted bread or lettuce wraps with tomatoes, bell peppers, and falafels.

Cure For The Garden: Featuring The Methionine Restriction Protocol   Copyright 2019. DocRhi.com

The Secret To Going Vegan Is In The Special Sauce!

Tahini Sauce

Blend all ingredients in a single serving blender cup until smooth, top with paprika and serve with roasted or fresh cauliflower, falafels, beets, or any other raw vegetable.

- 2 tablespoons tahini
- 2 tablespoons olive oil
- The juice of 1 lemon
- Sea salt to taste
- 1/3 cup water
- 1/2 teaspoon thyme
- 1/2 teaspoon sumac (optional)

The Secret To Going Vegan Is In The Special Sauce!

Sauces

Pesto

- 2 loose cups washed, fresh basil

- 2 tablespoons olive oil

- 2 tablespoons nutritional yeast

- The juice of 1 lemon

- 1/4 cup walnuts or pine nuts

- Sea salt to taste

- Water as needed

- 1 teaspoon garlic

- 1/2 teaspoon each oregano and rosemary (optional)

Blend all ingredients in a single serving blender cup until smooth. Serve atop steamed vegetables or lentil pasta.

Mexican Pesto

Blend all ingredients in a single serving blender cup until smooth. Serve atop steamed chayote squash (which has almost no Methionine), broccoli or other vegetable.

- 2 loose cups washed, fresh cilantro

- 2 tablespoons olive oil

- 2 tablespoons nutritional yeast

- The juice of 1 lime

- 1/4 cup walnuts or pine nuts

- Sea salt to taste

- Water as needed

- 1 teaspoon garlic

- 1/2 teaspoon each oregano, thyme and

The Secret To Going Vegan Is In The Special Sauce!

Vegan Mayonnaise

The development of this mayonnaise alone has completely changed our diet and digestion. Many vegan substitutions that are premade are full of oils that go rancid in transit and cause oxidation in our bodies (the chemical process that causes wrinkles and cancer). This mayo is plant based with no cooked oil and very little oil from the tahini.

- 1 cup drained, rinsed hearts of palm
- 1/4 cup water
- 2 tablespoons tahini
- 1 teaspoon sea salt
- Juice of 1 lemon
- 2 teaspoon white vinegar
- 1/2 teaspoon black pepper

Add all ingredients to high speed blender and process until smooth.

"This mayonnaise alone has completely changed our diet and digestion.."

Horseradish Sauce

Add 2 tablespoons extra-virgin olive oil, 2 teaspoons horseradish (or to taste), 1 teaspoon nutritional yeast to the above mayonnaise and blend. This sauce is wonderful on beets, squash and cauliflower steaks.

Creamy Taco Sauce

Add 2 tablespoons extra-virgin olive oil, finely chopped, 2 tablespoons de-seeded serrano chili, cilantro, chives, juice of 1 lime to the above mayonnaise and blend. This sauce is wonderful on tacos or as a fresh vegetable dip for parties.

Cure For The Garden: Featuring The Methionine Restriction Protocol   Copyright 2019. DocRhi.com

Sides, Snacks, and Apps

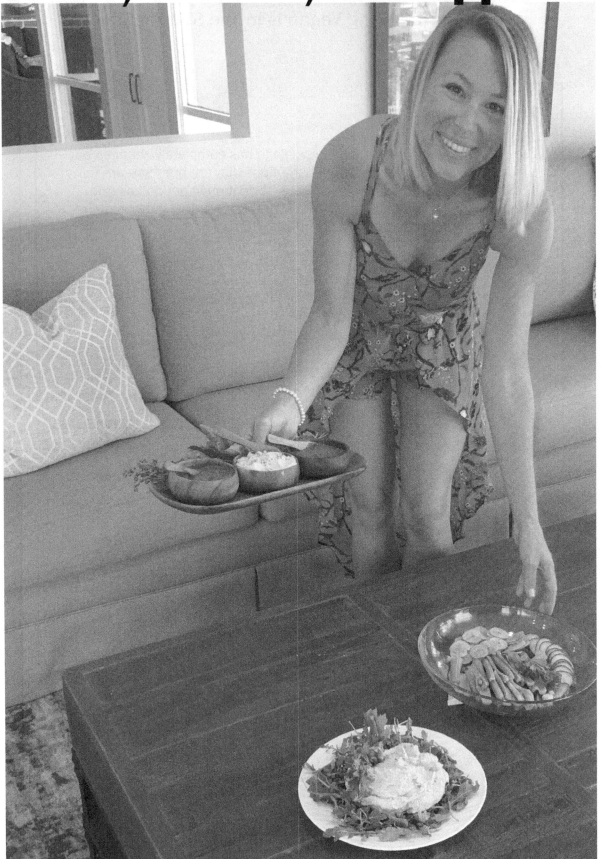

Having Many Dishes To Choose From Satiates Cravings!

Falafels

These falafels are great if you don't have time to completely sprout your lentils but only enough time to soak them the night before. Place all in a food processor. Blend on high until smooth, stirring occasionally. When you stir, scrape the sides. Pour enough oil into the skillet, using just enough to coat the bottom.

- 1/4 cup sesame seeds
- 1 cup chopped onions
- 1/2 cup chopped fresh parsley
- 1/8 cup fresh mint, or to taste
- 1/4 cup tahini
- 3 cups lentils, soaked overnight and drained of water (must be completely covered with water for overnight soaking)
- 5 crushed cloves fresh garlic, or to taste
- 1 teaspoon coriander
- 1 teaspoon cumin
- 1 teaspoon sea salt
- 1/2 teaspoon black pepper
- 1/2 teaspoon or less cayenne pepper
- 1 teaspoon paprika
- 1 tablespoon each flax meal and psyllium husk

Cook 1 flattened heaping teaspoon until golden brown, and then turn over on medium heat in pan or on the stove at 325F for 30 mins or until dry when a toothpick is inserted or dehydrate overnight.

Sides, Snacks, and Appetizers

Cure For The Garden: Featuring The Methionine Restriction Protocol   Copyright 2019. DocRhi.com

Having Many Dishes To Choose From Satiates Cravings!

Choose Your Spice Roasted Cauliflower

- 1/2 teaspoon each thyme, sumac, sesame, salt

- Or 1/2 teaspoon each cumin, coriander, paprika, salt

- Or 1/2 teaspoon each salt, sesame, dried onion, dried garlic, poppy seeds, caraway seeds

- 1 large cauliflower

Wash and cut cauliflower into small pieces, place all ingredients into a bag and shake. Lay out onto cookie sheet and bake at 425F for 30 minutes or until light golden.

Dip in Tahini Sauce!

Garbanzo Corn-nuts

Substitute cauliflower out for 1 can of garbanzo beans (or 1 cup home-cooked garbanzo beans) place all ingredients into a bag and shake. Lay out onto cookie sheet and bake at 325F for 60-90 minutes or until crunchy, turning every 30 minutes.

Sides, Snacks, and Appetizers

Cure For The Garden: Featuring The Methionine Restriction Protocol   Copyright 2019. DocRhi.com

Having Many Dishes To Choose From Satiates Cravings!

Sides, Snacks, and Appetizers

Potato Salad

Mix all ingredients in large salad bowl and top with paprika. Refrigerate 1 hour before serving.

- 4 large boiled or pressure cooked potatoes, cooled and cut into bite sized chunks
- 2 large stalks of celery, diced
- 1 small red or yellow onion diced
- 1 small green apple, diced
- 2 or 3 dill pickles
- 1 palm heart, sliced (optional)
- 1 teaspoon sea salt or to taste
- 2 tablespoon apple cider vinegar
- 1 teaspoon black pepper or to taste
- 2 tablespoons mustard or to taste
- 1 teaspoon dill
- 3 tablespoons Vegan Mayonnaise (See sauces)
- 1 teaspoon paprika

Pea Salad

For pea salad, substitute 2 cans of young peas (unsweetened) instead of the potatoes, 2 tablespoons of pimentos instead of the green apple and 3 tablespoons of vegan cheese shreds (we use vegan mozzarella) instead of the mustard!

Broccoli Slaw

For broccoli slaw, substitute 1 cup of shredded carrots, cabbage, and broccoli instead of the potatoes. To spice it up, you can optionally add 1/8 cup chopped peanuts and 1 de-seeded chopped jalapeño.

Having Many Dishes To Choose From Satiates Cravings!

Mexicali Slaw

Mix all ingredients in a large bowl. Let sit 15 minutes, mix again and serve.

- 1 1/2 cups of chopped green cabbage
- 1/4 of a red onion chopped
- 1/4 cup chopped peanuts
- 1/8 cup chopped cilantro
- 1 de-seeded, chopped Anaheim chili for mild or 2 de-seeded, chopped jalapenos for spicy slaw
- 2 tablespoon vegan mayo
- 1/2 tablespoon white vinegar
- 1/2 tablespoon lemon or lime juice
- sea salt to taste
- 1/2 teaspoon each black pepper, oregano, cumin
- 1 teaspoon minced garlic
- A pinch red chili powder (optional)

Cure For The Garden: Featuring The Methionine Restriction Protocol   Copyright 2019. DocRhi.com

Having Many Dishes To Choose From Satiates Cravings!

Sides, Snacks, and Appetizers

Quick Hummus

Drain 1 can of organic chick peas and place the contents of both cans (including the water of 1 of the cans) into blender. Add all other ingredients and blend on high until smooth. Pour into a bowl and garnish with paprika and zaatar (a Lebanese spice containing thyme, sesame and sumac) if you want and serve with veggies of any kind, we love the jicama!

This recipe is quick and simple especially if you have guests coming that you didn't plan for! To make red pepper hummus, chop and dry roast small sweet red peppers in a skillet for a few minutes and stir them in with the cayenne pepper.

- 2 cans of organic chick peas
- 1/8 cup tahini sauce (sesame paste)
- juice of 1 lemon
- 4 garlic cloves
- 2 tablespoons of olive oil
- 1/2 teaspoon coriander
- 1 teaspoon each of cumin and sea salt
- 1/8 teaspoon cayenne (optional)
- 1/4 teaspoon paprika & zaatar (optional)

Cure For The Garden: Featuring The Methionine Restriction Protocol   Copyright 2019. DocRhi.com

Having Many Dishes To Choose From Satiates Cravings!

Sprouted Lentil Hummus

Place all ingredients into high speed blender or food processor and mix until smooth and creamy. You may add a small amount of water if needed for creaminess (this will depend upon how much water your lentils have soaked up). Top with olive oil and paprika or sumac. Serve with carrot, celery, jicama, red bell pepper or any other vegetable sticks, and falafels.

Dehydrating conserves the enzymes in food and you can taste the difference! We highly recommend getting a dehydrator and to dehydrate your falafels, burger patties, fruit, veggie-chips, and crackers.

- 2 cups sprouted lentils
- 1/8 cup tahini
- 1 tablespoon minced garlic
- 2 tablespoons virgin olive oil
- 2 teaspoons coriander (we heap mine)
- 1 teaspoon cumin
- 1 teaspoon sea salt
- 1/8 teaspoon cayenne
- 1/8 cup lemon juice or more depending on your taste
- 1 teaspoon paprika or sumac to top hummus
- 1 tablespoon olive oil to drizzle

Sides, Snacks, and Appetizers

Cure For The Garden: Featuring The Methionine Restriction Protocol   Copyright 2019. DocRhi.com

Having Many Dishes To Choose From Satiates Cravings!

Sides, Snacks, and Appetizers

Baba Ghanoush

Preheat oven to 350.

Wash and prick the eggplant. Place onto baking sheet and bake 30-40 minutes until soft to touch and saggy. Cool to touch and peel. Place into food processor or high speed blender with all ingredients and blend until smooth. Serve topped with paprika and drizzled olive oil as a dip with falafel, cucumbers or romaine lettuce leaves.

- 1 eggplant
- 1/4 cup tahini
- 1/4 cup lemon juice or more to taste
- 2 tablespoons virgin olive oil
- 1 heaping tablespoon minced garlic
- 2 teaspoons coriander
- 1 teaspoon cumin
- 1 teaspoon sea salt
- 1 tablespoon sesame seeds
- 1 tablespoon homemade vegan mayo (see Sauces section) or tahini sauce
- 1 teaspoon paprika
- 1 teaspoon thyme (optional)

"Even people that think they don't like eggplant will love this .."

Cure For The Garden: Featuring The Methionine Restriction Protocol   Copyright 2019. DocRhi.com

Having Many Dishes To Choose From Satiates Cravings!

Green Olive Tapenade

- 1 tablespoon tomato paste
- 1 small can sliced mushrooms
- 1 large can of olives pitted
- 1 teaspoon sea salt
- 1 teaspoon Italian spices
- 1 teaspoon basil
- 1 teaspoon garlic
- 1/2 teaspoon dried onions

This recipe was invented by our good friend when she found out she had cancer. She immediately started the Methionine Restriction diet and is in remission!

In a small blender cup, mix 1/4 of the can of the olives and other ingredients except the olives. Chop remaining olives and add by hand to the mixed ingredients. Serve with vegetable sticks, flat bread and romaine leaves.

Sides, Snacks, and Appetizers

Cure For The Garden: Featuring The Methionine Restriction Protocol   Copyright 2019. DocRhi.com

Having Many Dishes To Choose From Satiates Cravings!

Gluten Free Bruschetta

Mix dry ingredients. Add 3/4 cup water. Stir for 2 minutes. If dough is stiff, add more water. Allow dough to sit for a couple of minutes so the flour can soak up some of the water then re-stir for a minute. Flatten onto an oiled cookie sheet.

Bake at 400F degrees for 28-30 minutes, until the top is golden.

Cut into rectangles and top with pesto, or marinara and veggies!

Makes a meal for 2-3 people or appetizers for 6-8.

- 2 cups yam, banana, or bean flour
- 1 cup nut or seed flour
- 1 teaspoon each baking powder and soda
- 1 teaspoon salt
- 1 tablespoon each psyllium husk and flax meal
- 3/4–1 cup sparkling water

Tips for switching any recipe to grain-free, no added oil, and egg-free:

Substitute flours for a blend of 2-3 parts yam, banana, or bean flour and 1 part nut flour. Use 1-2 tablespoons of psyllium husk and flax seed , 1 teaspoon of aluminum free baking soda and baking powder and after stirring together all of the other ingredients add very cold sparkling water instead of milk or regular water. This will cause the heavier flours to rise without needing the oil or egg.

Sides, Snacks, and Appetizers

Cure For The Garden: Featuring The Methionine Restriction Protocol   Copyright 2019. DocRhi.com

Having Many Dishes To Choose From Satiates Cravings!

Sides, Snacks, and Appetizers

Artichokes

Some people are afraid to cook artichokes because they have never cooked them before...they are really easy and so good for the liver. With a knife, cut the bottom stem off close to the bottom of the choke so that it stands up straight. Then cut off the top points of the choke. Next, with scissors trim off the points of the leaves. Place the choke in a covered saucepan with about an inch of water with 1 bag of orange pekoe or black tea. Simmer until leaves pull off very easily but watch to make sure to keep water in the pan so it doesn't burn, usually about 40 min. depending on the size of the chokes.

To serve, pull all leaves off and distribute in a circular fashion around the plate. Scrape the hairs from the top of the heart (center soft portion). Cut heart into wedges and place into center of plate or save for spinach-artichoke dip. Drizzle with olive oil, lemon juice, sea salt and garlic (optional) or dip in homemade vegan mayonnaise.

"Really easy and so good for the liver.."

- 3-4 artichokes
- 1 black tea or orange pekoe tea bag
- 1 tablespoon olive oil
- 1/2 tablespoon lemon juice
- 1/2 teaspoon sea salt
- 1/2 teaspoon dried or minced fresh garlic (optional)

Eat by scraping meat off of the leaves with your teeth. The inner leaves and heart can just be eaten. Enjoy! we make 1 for each person or 1 for 2 people to share if we am serving it with other things.

Cure For The Garden: Featuring The Methionine Restriction Protocol   Copyright 2019. DocRhi.com

Having Many Dishes To Choose From Satiates Cravings!

Vegan Artichoke and Spinach Dip

- 4 artichoke hearts
- 1 cup fresh spinach leaves
- 1/2 vegan cheese shreds
- 1/2 cup vegan homemade parmesan cheese
- 1/2 cup vegan mayo
- 1 tablespoons minced garlic
- 1 teaspoon sea salt
- 1 and 1/2 tablespoons lemon juice

Place spinach leaves into food processor and pulse. Add all other ingredients and pulse until mixed but not smooth. Pour into pan and top with vegan parmesan. Bake at 400 F for 20-30 minutes and until light brown. Serve with vegetable sticks such as jicama, carrots, celery and cucumber.

Vegan Parmesan Cheese

- 1/2 cup nutritional yeast
- 1/4 cup roasted almonds
- 1 tablespoon dried ground shitake mushrooms
- 1 teaspoon sea salt
- 2 teaspoon Italian spices (optional)

Place all ingredients into high speed blender. Make sure your blender is very dry so your vegan parmesan doesn't get wet! Mix thoroughly and use as any other ground parmesan cheese.

Sides, Snacks, and Appetizers

Having Many Dishes To Choose From Satiates Cravings!

Marinated Red Onions

Thinly slice red onion and place into jar. Add spices and fill with white vinegar. Close jar and place into refrigerator for at least 3 days. The onion will stay good for a long time if covered in vinegar in the refrigerator. Serve on salads, veggie tacos, veggie fajitas, and to spice up other dishes. It turns a beautiful pink.

You can also marinate radishes or turnips using the same recipe!

- 1 small red onion
- white vinegar
- 2 teaspoon dried oregano
- 1 teaspoon sea salt
- 1 teaspoon black pepper
- 1 recycled mason jar

"Serve on salads, veggie tacos, veggie fajitas, and to spice up other dishes.

Sides, Snacks, and Appetizers

Cure For The Garden: Featuring The Methionine Restriction Protocol   Copyright 2019. DocRhi.com

Having Many Dishes To Choose From Satiates Cravings!

Curried Veggies

In a hot pan, add water, potatoes or cauliflower, garlic and ginger. Mix, cover and sauté until soft but not mushy. Add all other ingredients and sea salt to taste and let sit 2 or 3 hours in the refrigerator. Serve chilled.

- 1 cup of chopped cauliflower or chopped potatoes
- 1 tablespoon extra virgin olive oil
- Juice of two lemons
- 1/8 cup water
- 1/2 cup shredded carrots
- 1/2 cup diced red bell pepper
- 1/4 cup scallions or green onions
- 1 small tomato diced
- 1 teaspoon curry powder
- 1 teaspoon crushed garlic
- 1 teaspoon crushed or dried ginger
- 1/2 cup green peas (optional)

Cure For The Garden: Featuring The Methionine Restriction Protocol   Copyright 2019. DocRhi.com

Sides, Snacks, and Appetizers

Entrees

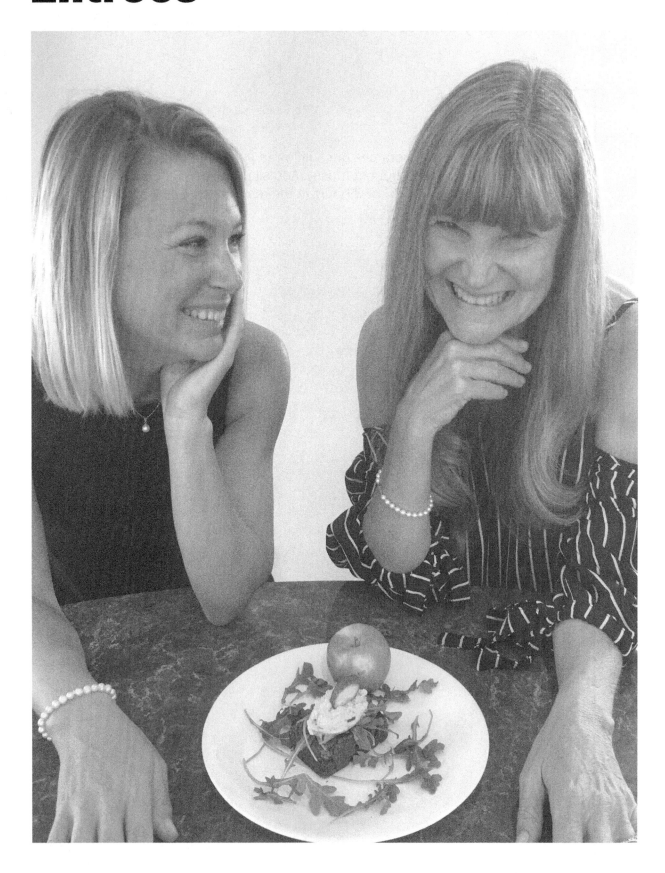

Cure For The Garden: Featuring The Methionine Restriction Protocol

Entrees, The Main Event!

Pizza For Breakfast, Lunch, Snack or Dinner? When food tastes this good and is this good for you, there is no reason not to eat it any time of day! You can interchange the spices with bagel spices such as salt, caraway seeds, black and white sesame seeds and use onions, garlic and broccoli or zucchini or yellow squash, throw some bell pepper on top and you've got a great treat for mornings that refrigerates and freezes well. We like to make one of these almost every other day because they only take about 10 minutes to put together and are so satisfying.

Pizza

Preheat your oven to 325F. Mix the flour, salt and water together slowly in a bowl, stirring continuously and allowing the flour to

- 2 cups garbanzo bean/ chickpea flour

- 1/2– 3/4 cup of sparkling water

- 2 cups of veggies such as onions, artichokes, pitted olives, zucchini, tomato, bell pepper etc. or you may use premade olive or artichoke tapenade

- 1/2 teaspoon of each salt, baking soda, and powder, garlic powder, rosemary, basil, thyme, fennel seed, parsley

- 1-2 tablespoons of toppings such as nutritional yeast, red pepper flakes, basil

"Pizza For Breakfast, Lunch, Snack or Dinner? They only take about 10 minutes to put together.."

absorb the water before adding more. The mixture should be a toothpaste consistency.

Mix vegetables and spices right into the dough. Press the mixture thin into a large cast iron skillet that has been oiled and floured and bake for 30-60 minutes (depending upon thickness) at 325F or until lightly browned. Use toppings of choice. Dip in Noni Blue Cheese Dressing!

Entrees, The Main Event!

Double Stuffed Potatoes

Preheat oven to 425 F. Wash, rub with sea salt and prick potatoes. Bake until fork enters easily, but not mushy. Let cool.

In hot sauté pan, add water onions, garlic, mushrooms and kale. Cook until kale is bright green. Remove from heat. With spoon, scrape out flesh of potato into sauté pan, leaving some to keep sides firm. Lightly mix with all other ingredients in sauté pan for 5 minutes at medium heat, crushing potato and other ingredients together. Spoon mixture back into potato skins.

- 4 potatoes (We like to use purple Okanogan potatoes)
- 4 green onions chopped
- 1 tablespoon crushed garlic
- 1 cup kale or spinach chopped small
- 2 tablespoons water
- 1/2 cup chopped white mushrooms (optional)
- 1 teaspoon sea salt
- 1 teaspoon black pepper
- 1 teaspoon paprika
- 1/4 cup of vegan cheese shreds
- 1 tablespoon vegan parmesan
- 1 teaspoon parsley flakes (optional)

Top with vegan cheese shreds, vegan parmesan and paprika. Bake for 10 minutes or until cheese is melted and golden. Serve with an arugula salad!

Entrees, The Main Event!

This healthy mac-n-cheese made this diet possible for us. Our ancestors were from the south where it is a big tradition. So we think having this comfort food is a necessity!

- 3 tablespoons homemade vegan mayo (See Sauces section)
- 2 tablespoons olive oil
- 4 teaspoons nutritional yeast or homemade vegan parmesan (See Sauces section)
- 1/2 teaspoon garlic powder
- Salt and pepper to taste

Healthy Mac-N-Cheese

Make lentil noodles as directed on package (we use elbow noodles/ sedanini red lentil noodles). Remove from heat, drain through a colander and rinse with hot water.

Stir all remaining ingredients into noodles and serve.

"Our ancestors were from the south where it is a big tradition..."

Switching this recipe up for other pastas is quite easy! Try this one!

Artichoke Linguini

Make lentil or edamame noodles as directed on package (we like Non-GMO edamame noodles from Asian markets). In a saucepan on low heat, stir in 4 tablespoons of the homemade Vegan Mayonnaise, 5 teaspoons of the homemade Vegan Parmesan, 1/4 cup chopped mushrooms, 1/2 cup drained artichoke hearts (optional), 1 teaspoon each of oregano, dried garlic and onion powder, 1 1/2 teaspoons basil, 1/2 teaspoon thyme, rosemary and fennel. Heat and serve over noodles.

Cure For The Garden: Featuring The Methionine Restriction Protocol   Copyright 2019. DocRhi.com

Entrees, The Main Event!

This dish is really great for parties and food prepping for the week. Try it on the Pumpkin Beer Bread with avocado and sprouts and you won't feel like you are missing out on a thing!

Vegan Tuna Salad

Soak 1 1/2 cups sunflower seeds overnight and drain off water. Place in a high speed blender and add all other ingredients except celery, onion and pickles. Blend on high until well mixed then hand mix in all other ingredients. Enjoy immediately or refrigerate for sandwiches!

- 1 1/2 cup soaked sunflower seeds
- 2 tablespoons homemade vegan mayo (See Sauces section)
- 1/8 cup dried wakame seaweed (other seaweeds like nori are not quite as good)
- 1 tablespoon pickle juice
- 1 tablespoon capers
- 1 teaspoon coconut aminos
- 1/4 cup chopped onion
- 1 cup chopped celery
- 1/4 cup chopped pickles
- Salt and pepper to taste
- 1/2 teaspoon fennel seed (optional)

"Try it on the Pumpkin Beer Bread with avocado and sprouts..."

Entrees, The Main Event!

Squash Steaks

Cut a squash in half, remove the seeds and place face down in a baking pan with 1/2-inch of water in the bottom of pan. Bake at 325 for 30 minutes or until the squash has a slight give but is still firm when pressed with a spoon. Allow the squash to cool then cut 2-inch steaks from the squash. Put all other ingredients into a skillet, allow the herbs and vinegar to cook for 3 minutes, stirring occasionally then add squash steaks and mushrooms. Cook at medium heat for 10 minutes and flip steaks to the other side when golden.

- 2-inch squash steaks (butternut or other) from a squash that has been roasted in the oven until it gives slightly when pressed with a spoon but still firm

- Sliced mushrooms

- 1/8 cup balsamic

- 1/8 cup coconut aminos

- 1/8 cup water

- 1/2 teaspoon salt

- 1 teaspoon each thyme, rosemary, sage, parsley, onion, garlic

"Top with horseradish sauce for a gourmet culinary experience..."

Top with kale and cover and cook for another 10 minutes, or until the bottom side of steaks achieve the golden brown color on both sides. Top with horseradish sauce for a gourmet culinary experience.

Cure For The Garden: Featuring The Methionine Restriction Protocol   Copyright 2019. DocRhi.com

Entrees, The Main Event!

Entrees

Red Potatoes and Greens

Place 1/4 cup water and salt in a non-stick pan at medium heat. Lay potatoes face down in the bottom of pan, cover and simmer for 10-15 minutes, stirring occasionally. Add greens and more water if the water has cooked off and stir. Cover and cook 5 more minutes or until greens are a brighter color.

Top with pepper and smoked paprika.

- 2 cups red potatoes, sliced lengthwise
- 3 cups greens (chard, kale, collards, mustard)
- 1/8 cup balsamic
- 1/8 cup coconut aminos
- 1/4– 1/2 cup water
- 1/2 teaspoon salt, pepper, smoked paprika
- 1 teaspoon each onion and garlic, fresh or powder

"Try beans or black eyed peas instead of potatoes..."

You can also try beans or black eyed peas instead of potatoes. We like to prepare a meal with potatoes and greens as well as beans with a different type of seasonal green.

Cure For The Garden: Featuring The Methionine Restriction Protocol   Copyright 2019. DocRhi.com

Entrees, The Main Event!

Entrees

Vegetable Fajitas

- 1 each: red, yellow, green, and bell pepper, de-seeded and sliced lengthwise
- 1 large pasilla chili, sliced thin, de-seeded
- 1 large red onion, sliced thinly
- 1/2 cup each sliced mushrooms and broccoli
- 2 large roma tomatoes, sliced thinly lengthwise
- 3 tomatillos, sliced lengthwise
- 1 large jalapeno, completely de-seeded and chopped small
- 1/4 cup fresh cilantro
- 1/8 cup fresh oregano
- Sea salt to taste
- 1 teaspoon dried cumin
- 3 tablespoons water
- 2 chopped garlic cloves

Heat the water in a skillet. Sauté vegetables and garlic until tender, but still firm. Add spices, fresh cilantro and the juice of one lemon. Serve with cabbage leaves. Lastly, top with guacamole. Serves 4. Optionally, use half of the vegetables and save the other half for enchilada soup.

"Start cooking your firmer veggies first or cut firmer vegies thinner to achieve a soft yet snappy vegetable consistency throughout..."

You can optionally add other vegetables as well! When you are sautéing vegetables, the consistency is more even throughout when you start with firmer vegies or cut firmer vegies thinner. For example, start with thin sliced onion and chilis on the bottom, after 1 minute add thinly sliced carrots and potatoes then add broccoli, zucchini, squash and mushrooms.

Cure For The Garden: Featuring The Methionine Restriction Protocol   Copyright 2019. DocRhi.com

Entrees, The Main Event!

Nut Burgers

Beat in a food processor until thoroughly mixed and holds together well. Let stand at room temperature for 1-2 hours. Dehydrate overnight, flipping once. Or, lightly coat a skillet with olive oil, heat pan on medium heat and drop mixture by heaping tablespoons into hot pan. Cook until lightly brown on edges, turn and press flat into patties. Cook until golden brown and turn one more time.

- 1 small brown onion
- 1 cup cashews
- 1 cup sprouted lentils
- 1 cup yam or plantain flour
- 1 tablespoon psyllium husk
- 1 tablespoon ground flax seed
- 1 1/2 tablespoons balsamic vinegar
- 1 1/2 tablespoons tamari or coconut aminos
- 5 cloves fresh crushed garlic
- 1/4 teaspoon cayenne pepper
- 1/4 teaspoon black pepper
- 1/4 teaspoon white pepper
- 1 teaspoon cumin
- 1 teaspoon oregano

"An easy freeze for dinners down the road.."

Serve on lettuce wraps with favorite garnishes. The nut burgers make a great easy freeze for dinners down the road! Optionally, you can roll patties in onion flakes prior to dehydrating or cooking.

Cure For The Garden: Featuring The Methionine Restriction Protocol   Copyright 2019. DocRhi.com

Entrees, The Main Event!

Sprouted Organic Tofu Burgers

Squeeze all of the water out of the tofu by squeezing it through a cheesecloth. Blend all contents in food processor and let sit 1 hour. Spoon dough onto a nonstick griddle and cook on medium heat until golden, flip and flatten, flip and flatten again. Serve or let cool and crumble and use as any ground meat . We like to reuse by adding to spaghetti or tacos!

- 16 oz. Sprouted firm tofu (organic, watch out for GMO)
- 1 cup yam or plantain flour
- 1 tablespoon psyllium husk
- 1 tablespoon ground flax seed
- 1/2 yellow onion
- 2 tablespoons organic tomato paste
- 3 cloves of garlic
- 1 tablespoons balsamic vinegar
- 1 teaspoon cumin
- 1/2 teaspoon each oregano and sea salt
- 1/8 teaspoon cayenne
- 1/2 cup juicing leftover shreds, food-processed well

"Reuse by adding to spaghetti or tacos!.."

An optional spin is to dehydrate your patties overnight or boil patties in 1/8 cup water with 1 teaspoon powdered shitake mushrooms (grind yourself in a high speed blender), and 1 teaspoon each garlic and onion powder.

Cure For The Garden: Featuring The Methionine Restriction Protocol   Copyright 2019. DocRhi.com

Entrees, The Main Event!

Spaghetti Squash and Marinara

Pre heat oven to 400F degrees.

- 1 spaghetti squash
- 5 large tomatoes or 1 large can of organic chopped tomatoes
- 2 stocks of chopped celery
- 1 small white onion chopped
- 1 red bell pepper chopped
- 1 cup chopped mushrooms (white or brown)
- 1 cup kale leaves
- 1 tablespoon minced garlic or more depending on taste
- 1 tablespoon balsamic vinegar
- pinch of stevia leaves
- 1 teaspoon sea salt
- 2 teaspoon dried basil or 4 tablespoons of fresh
- 1 teaspoon each of dried oregano, thyme, parsley, rosemary and fennel seeds
- 2 tablespoons water

Cut the spaghetti squash in half length-wise, remove seeds and place open side down into glass casserole pan. Add 2 inches of water and bake until a knife goes into the squash easily.

While squash is cooking, place the water, onions, celery, and pepper into a hot skillet on medium heat water.

Entrees, The Main Event!

Spaghetti Squash and Marinara

Cook until onions are transparent. Add garlic, mushrooms and kale with vinegar, stevia, spices and salt. Mix well and add tomatoes. Lower heat and sauté for about 30 minutes. Serve with spaghetti squash, zucchini noodles, mung noodles, on flat bread pizzas and eggplant. Top with vegan parmesan.
over.

Take spaghetti squash out of oven and let cool for a few minutes until you are able to touch it. Use a fork to scrape the meat of the squash down to the peel, scrapping all of the meat out in long strips. Place in serving bowl and spoon the marinara over. Garnish with fresh basil and serve with a green salad.

Garnish with fresh basil and serve with a green salad.

Entrees, The Main Event!

Pesto Vegetables

Mix all ingredients in blender until smooth and serve on spaghetti squash, zucchini sticks steamed or raw, or in a lettuce wrap.

For a Mexican Pesto twist, substitute cilantro for the basil and add green onion, cumin, oregano, juice of 1 lemon, and cayenne and you have cilantro pesto which is great mixed with steamed Mexican (chayote) squash or fresh salad as a dressing.

- 1 1/2 cups of fresh chopped basil
- 1/2 cup pine nuts (walnuts or try any nut / seed you like)
- 1/3 cup grated vegan cheese or 3-4 teaspoons nutritional yeast
- 5 cloves of garlic
- 1/2 cup of olive oil
- Sea salt to taste

"For a Mexican Pesto twist, substitute cilantro .."

Cure For The Garden: Featuring The Methionine Restriction Protocol

Copyright 2019. DocRhi.com

Entrees, The Main Event!

Stuffed Mushrooms

Bring water to a boil in a small saucepan. Add walnuts and cook until they have softened slightly, about 5 minutes. Drain and set aside. With same water, sauté mushrooms and stems. Drain and chop stems. Combine stems, rosemary and 1 pinch sea salt in the bowl of a mortar and pestle, food processor, or high-speed blender and add walnuts, marjoram, thyme, basil and oregano. Pulse the blender and grind until combined and slightly creamy, but still coarse. Transfer the walnut mixture to a large bowl. Slowly whisk in olive oil to form a thick emulsion. Add smashed avocados and whip. Season with black pepper and sea salt to taste. Stuff walnut sauce into mushroom caps.

- 1 cups water, or as needed
- 1 1/2 cups walnuts
- 3 large avocados
- 1 pinch sea salt
- 1 teaspoon chopped fresh marjoram
- 1 teaspoon chopped fresh thyme
- 1 teaspoon chopped fresh oregano
- 1/2 cup extra-virgin olive oil freshly ground black
- pepper to taste
- sea salt to taste
- 1/2 teaspoon fennel seeds
- 1 1/2 cups shitake mushrooms, stemmed (save stems)

Garnish with fennel seeds. Serve with finely chopped and crushed baby kale.

Cure For The Garden: Featuring The Methionine Restriction Protocol   Copyright 2019. DocRhi.com

Entrees, The Main Event!

Eggplant Parmesan

Preheat oven to 350 F. Wash eggplant, thinly slice and lightly salt it. Mix flax meal with 1 tablespoon of Vegan Parmesan Cheese (See Recipe), salt and Italian spices, and place in flat dish. Place milk into flat dish. Dip eggplant one at a time into the nut milk and then into the flax mixture. Place onto non-stick baking sheet and bake for 20 minutes. Turn and bake until light brown.

Layer eggplant into 4 stacks in this order: eggplant, marinara, vegan cheese shreds, parmesan until all of the eggplant is used. Bake covered for about 30 minutes until cheese is melted and marinara is bubbly, being careful not to burn.

- 1 eggplant
- 1/2 cup vegan parmesan cheese
- 1/2 cup vegan mozzarella cheese shreds
- 1/2 cup of almond or hemp milk
- 2 tablespoons of flax meal
- 2 teaspoons of Italian spices (see spice it right page)
- 1 teaspoon sea salt
- 1/4 cup nut milk

Cure For The Garden: Featuring The Methionine Restriction Protocol   Copyright 2019. DocRhi.com

Entrees, The Main Event!

Roasted Eggplant

Preheat oven to 375 F.

Wash eggplant, cut into cubes and lay out on flat dish. Salt each piece and let sit for at least 2 hours. Rinse eggplant in colander and pat dry. Mix all dressing ingredients in cup high speed blender. Mix thoroughly with eggplant cubes and spread in one layer on a non-stick baking sheet. Bake for 20 minutes and turn. Bake for another 15 minutes or until light brown and crispy.

Serve as a side dish, entrée or appetizer.

- 1 eggplant
- 1 red bell pepper
- 1 small red onion
- Dressing
- 1 teaspoon orange peel
- 1 orange peeled, separated and cut into halves.
- 1 teaspoon minced garlic
- 1 teaspoon minced ginger
- 2 tablespoons chopped fresh Thai basil
- 1/2 teaspoon white pepper
- 1/8 cup sea salt

Entrees, The Main Event!

Breaded Zucchini

In a large bowl, combine flax, psyllium and flour, then mix in nut milk and allow mixture to sit out for 1 hour.

Preheat oven to 375 F.

Wash zucchini and slice thinly at a diagonal to make longer. Mix spices and parmesan into flour mixture. Dip zucchini into breading mixture, making sure they are completely coated with breading. Place on a non-stick baking sheet and bake for 15 minutes. Turn and bake until crispy, about 15 minutes more. Serve hot with veggie marinara or top with vegan shredded cheese.

- 1 medium zucchini (large is too woody)
- 1 cup homemade nut or tahini milk
- 1/2 cup vegan parmesan
- 1 tablespoon flax meal
- 1 tablespoon psyllium husk
- 1/4 cup water chestnut or yam flour
- 1 teaspoon sea salt
- 2 teaspoon Italian spices

Entrees, The Main Event!

Sweet Potato Gnocchi

Place all ingredients in a food processor and process until mixture balls up in the center of the food processor. Allow mixture to rest for 30 minutes. Add water a little at a time until you are able to roll the dough into snake like noodles and pinch off gnocchi 1-inch at a time. Let gnocchi pieces stand at room temperature for 1 hour.

Bring water to a boil in a small saucepan. Add sea salt to boiling water, toss in gnocchi pieces, turn over once with a spoon and remove when it floats to the top.

Serve with vegan parmesan cheese, veggie marinara, vegan pesto or fresh garlic with Italian spices, sea salt and olive oil.

- 2 cooked medium sweet potatoes
- 1 tablespoon flax seed meal
- 1 tablespoon psyllium husks
- 1 cup yam, lentil or bean flour
- 1 teaspoon sea salt
- 1/2 teaspoon black pepper
- 1 tablespoon minced garlic
- 1 teaspoon dried basil or 2 tablespoons fresh minced basil
- 1/2 teaspoon dried thyme or 1 teaspoon fresh minced thyme
- 1 teaspoon rosemary
- 1 teaspoon dried oregano or 1 tablespoon minced fresh oregano

Entrees, The Main Event!

Not– So Fried Okra

Dry roast pecans 10 minutes on medium heat, stirring occasionally. Toss pecans in with flour, salt and pepper. In another bowl wet chopped okra with water before pouring in pecan mixture. Press the mixture onto the okra pieces and cook for 5-6 minutes in a pan on medium heat. If tofu is desired press it into the pecan mixture and cook until golden. So simple and so good!

- 1/4 cup pecans

- 2 cups okra

- 1/2 cup banana or yam flour

- 1/2 teaspoon each of salt and pepper

- Non-GMO tofu cut in squares (optional)

- 1/4 cup water

Unless we absolutely cannot avoid it, we always want to use water, vinegar, tamari, coconut aminos or another water based sauce to cook our food in, and then add a little uncooked virgin oil after cooking. Heating oils results in toxins than are carcinogenic, or cancer causing!

Cure For The Garden: Featuring The Methionine Restriction Protocol   Copyright 2019. DocRhi.com

Entrees, The Main Event!

Sprouted Lentil Falafels

Place all ingredients in food processor and blend until smooth, stopping every couple of minutes to scrape the sides of the food processor. Form your falafels by hand into 1 inch balls and flatten, keeping them a uniform size. They can be baked at 375 F for 15 minutes and flip. Bake until golden, grilled on both sides until golden, or dehydrated. Dehydrated is my favorite!

- 2 cups of sprouted lentils
- 1/8 cup of sesame seeds (optional)
- 1/4 cup shopped fresh parsley
- 1/8 cup tahini
- 1/2 chopped onion
- 1 tablespoon minced garlic
- 2 heaping teaspoons coriander
- 1 heaping teaspoon cumin
- 1 teaspoon sea salt
- 1/2 teaspoon black pepper
- 1/4 teaspoon cayenne
- 1 teaspoon paprika or sumac
- 1/2 tablespoon lemon juice
- 1 tablespoon flax meal
- 1 tablespoon psyllium husk

Cure For The Garden: Featuring The Methionine Restriction Protocol   Copyright 2019. DocRhi.com

Entrees, The Main Event!

Sprouted Lentil Vegan Quiche Cups

Place the Sprouted Lentil Flatbread dough (See Baked Goods section) into non-stick, papered or oiled and floured muffin pan and bake at 375 F until light golden. Remove from oven.

Add 2 tablespoons water to skillet and warm over medium heat. When hot add salt, onions and spices. Cook a few minutes to mix tasted and add wrung out tofu (literally wrap a cloth around a block of tofu and wring out all of the water). Mix lightly, cover and let heat for a few minutes. Add spinach, mix lightly and cover. Cook until spinach is bright green.

- 1 package of non-GMO tofu (we use sprouted if we can find it)
- 1/4 chopped green onion
- 1/2 cup chopped sweet red peppers
- 2 cups fresh spinach
- 1 tablespoon garlic (optional)
- 1/4 cup vegan parmesan or vegan cheese shreds (optional)
- 1 teaspoon sea salt
- 1 teaspoon mustard powder
- 1/2 teaspoon red chili flakes or cumin
- water as needed to make sure the pan is slightly wet while cooking (so food doesn't stick)
- 1/2 cup chopped mushrooms (optional)

Spoon into each flatbread in the muffin pan and top with vegan parmesan or vegan cheese shreds and bake for 10 minutes at 350 F. Let cool and serve, or freeze for lunches, breakfasts, appetizers, snacks or when company comes.

Cure For The Garden: Featuring The Methionine Restriction Protocol   Copyright 2019. DocRhi.com

Eat The Warm With The Raw!

Once you get started, salad dressings are incredibly easy to make. Simply put all ingredients in a high speed blender and mix until smooth.

Vegan Blue Cheese Dressing

- 2 tablespoons virgin oil
- 2-inch by 4-inch square of noni leather (order online; it is grown in Hawaii)
- 2 tablespoons lemon juice
- 1/2 teaspoon sea salt
- 1/2 teaspoon black pepper
- 1 teaspoon garlic
- 1 teaspoon dill
- 2 tablespoons vegan mayo

Cut up noni leather with scissors and place into olive oil to dissolve and let sit for a few minutes. Place all ingredients into cup high speed blender. Serve over salad or as a dip for celery. Add more vegan mayo if thicker dip wanted.

Sesame Citrus Dressing

- 1/8 cup red wine vinegar
- 1/8 cup olive oil
- 1 teaspoon sea salt
- 1 teaspoon black pepper
- 1 teaspoon mustard powder
- 1 teaspoon zest of orange
- optional pinch of stevia leaves
- 1 tablespoon sesame seeds

Place all ingredients except sesame seeds into a high speed blender. Serve over salad topped with sesame seeds.

Salad Dressings

Cure For The Garden: Featuring The Methionine Restriction Protocol   Copyright 2019. DocRhi.com

Eat The Warm With The Raw!

Now try blending up your own! Here are some of our favorites!

Italian Salad Dressing

Olive oil, balsamic vinegar, fresh garlic and Italian seasonings like basil, oregano, rosemary, and fennel seed. If you add Dijon mustard, you have a really rich, spicy flavor. Good served with herbs and bitter greens, pine nuts or walnuts, and olives.

Mexican Salad Dressing

An avocado smashed with garlic, sea salt, oregano, chili powder, cumin, and lemon or lime juice is really good on a salad of chopped cabbage, tomatoes, bell peppers, brown onion, green chilies without the seeds, and cilantro.

Mediterranean Salad Dressing

Hummus (see Sides section) with extra lemon juice, sea salt, cumin, coriander, paprika, and olive oil is great on a salad of romaine, cucumbers, tomatoes, parsley, red onion, and sesame seeds.

If you are eating out at a restaurant ask for lemon, avocado and salt to use as a salad dressing or a dressing for steamed vegetables!

Eat The Warm With The Raw!

Two-bolli Salad

Wash and chop all veggies finely. In a large bowl, pour in the lemon juice, olive oil and salt over veggies and mix. Let stand for 45 minutes. Enjoy alone or with hummus, falafels, masala veggies, or lentil soup. This is great served in a lettuce wrap.

- two large tomatoes and their juice
- two large cucumbers
- two green onions
- two bunches of parsley
- two large lemons, juiced
- 1/2 cup olive oil
- A dash of sea salt & garlic to taste
- 1 cup cauliflower rice (frozen, then defrosted at room temperature for 2-3 hours for texture!)

Cure For The Garden: Featuring The Methionine Restriction Protocol   Copyright 2019. DocRhi.com

Eat The Warm With The Raw!

Baby Kale Salad with Faux Blue Cheese Dressing

The blue cheese dressing in this salad is not only amazing tasting but is also anti-cancer! You will immediately feel the energy in this salad when you eat it and can drench it in this dressing without worry! Wash and dry kale, tomatoes and cucumber before cutting. Add all ingredients into large bowl and pour dressing over. Top with optional vegan parmesan and toss. Serve as side dish or lunch.

Makes one entre or 2-3 side salads!

- 2 cups baby kale leaves
- 1 cup of cherry tomatoes halved
- 1 cucumber diced
- Blue Cheese dressing (See Dressings)
- Toasted cubes of Sweet Potato Bread (See Baked Goods) (optional)
- 1 tablespoon capers (optional)

"This dressing is not only amazing tasting but is also anti-cancer..."

Soups & Salads

Cure For The Garden: Featuring The Methionine Restriction Protocol   Copyright 2019. DocRhi.com

Eat The Warm With The Raw!

Soups & Salads

Kale Citrus Salad

Mix all ingredients in a large bowl and allow to chill for at least 2 hours before serving if you use large kale leaves so that the dressing can soften them. If you are using baby kale, you do not need to chill ahead of time.

Makes one entre or 2-3 side salads!

- 2 cups chopped, washed kale with stems removed or baby kale

- 1 orange, peeled, sectioned and cut in halves

- 1/2 cup marinated red onions (See Sides)

- Sesame Citrus dressing (See Salad Dressing section)

Cure For The Garden: Featuring The Methionine Restriction Protocol   Copyright 2019. DocRhi.com

Eat The Warm With The Raw!

Sprouted Lentil Salad

Place all ingredients into bowl and toss until well mixed, cover and place into refrigerator for at least 2 hours before serving. You can make this salad the night before serving. This is an excellent main dish during the summer time!

- 1 chopped zucchini
- 1 chopped tomato
- 1 cup sprouted lentils
- 1/2 cup chopped red onions
- 1/8 cup virgin olive oil
- 1/2 cup red wine vinegar
- 2 tablespoons lemon juice
- 2 teaspoons basil
- 1 teaspoon oregano
- 1 teaspoon rosemary
- 1/2 teaspoon fennel
- 1 teaspoon sea salt
- 1/2 teaspoon black pepper

Eat The Warm With The Raw!

Soups & Salads

Mango Beet Salad

In Eastern medicine beets help build blood cells! So, for vegan diets they are important. Each portion of an herb or food has slightly different qualities, so eat the whole beet including the "tail". The tail would have a more moving quality to improve blood circulation whereas the "body" of the beet would be more blood building.

Wash and quarter a large beet, place it on a non-stick cookie sheet, cover with water and a dash of salt and pepper, and bake uncovered for 40-50 minutes at 375F degrees. The beet will be fairly easy to cut when it is ready.

Cut up 1 large mango, 1 avocado, and beet greens. Top with 1 teaspoon of olive oil, the juice of ½ a lemon, a heaping tablespoon of coconut shavings,

- 1 large mango
- 1 avocado
- 4 cups cut beet greens
- 1 teaspoon of olive oil
- Juice of 1/2 a lemon
- 1 heaping tablespoon of coconut shavings
- 1/4 cup water
- A dash of salt and pepper

"Beets help build blood cells..."

and a dash of salt and pepper.

Makes one entre or 2-3 side salads!

You can also substitute out the beets for baked squash, such as butternut or acorn.

Cure For The Garden: Featuring The Methionine Restriction Protocol

Eat The Warm With The Raw!

Soups & Salads

Enchilada Soup

Preheat a skillet until hot on medium heat. Add water, carrots, onion, squash and spices and cook for a few minutes before adding all other ingredients. Stir mixture. Cover and simmer on low heat for one hour, stirring every 15 minutes.

Garnish with cilantro and serve with a slice of lime.

- 2 tablespoons water
- 1/2 the vegetables from the Vegetable Fajitas recipe
- 1/2 head of cabbage, chopped
- 4 carrots, thinly chopped
- 2 yellow or one acorn squash, finely chopped
- 1 cup enchilada sauce
- 4 cups water
- 5 cloves of crushed garlic
- 1 1/2 teaspoon cumin
- Juice of 1 lemon
- 1/2 teaspoon black pepper
- 1 can sliced black olives
- 1 teaspoon oregano
- 1 onion, finely chopped

Cure For The Garden: Featuring The Methionine Restriction Protocol   Copyright 2019. DocRhi.com

Eat The Warm With The Raw!

Soups & Salads

Lentil Dal Stew

Place 2 tablespoons of water in warm sauce pan and add onions. Cook until transparent. Add sprouted lentils, jalapeno, spices, garlic, carrots, zucchini, and celery and stir until spices coat everything. Add water and simmer on low for 40-45 minutes watching to make sure you have enough water.

- 2 cups of sprouted lentils
- 1/2 cup chopped onion
- 1 heaping tablespoon minced garlic
- 1 chopped zucchini
- 2 chopped carrots
- 2 chopped celery stalks
- 1 deseeded, chopped jalapeno
- 2 teaspoon coriander
- 1 teaspoon cumin
- 1/2 teaspoon thyme
- 1 teaspoon sesame seed
- 1/2 teaspoon black pepper
- 1/2 teaspoon cinnamon
- 1 teaspoon each sea salt and hing
- 2 tablespoons lemon juice
- 2 tablespoons chopped fresh cilantro

Tips for cooking with beans:

- Soak beans overnight and rinse the water before cooking.

- Use a pressure cooker for faster results and to breakdown the phytonutrient, Lignans, that can cause gas.

- Add the Indian spice called hing/asafetida.

Top with sesame seeds and cilantro, and serve as a first course or meal.

Cure For The Garden: Featuring The Methionine Restriction Protocol   Copyright 2019. DocRhi.com

Eat The Warm With The Raw!

Vegan Soup Stock

This is a great substitute for bouillon cubes. Grind all ingredient in cup high speed blender and keep in jar for use. Add 2-3 tablespoons of powder to a quart sauce pan for a stock.

- 1 cup dried shitake mushrooms
- 1 tablespoon dried garlic
- 2 tablespoons dried onions
- optional sea salt
- 1 teaspoon sesame seeds
- 1 teaspoon rosemary
- 1 teaspoon thyme

"Substitute for bouillon cubes..."

Soups & Salads

Cure For The Garden: Featuring The Methionine Restriction Protocol   Copyright 2019. DocRhi.com

Eat The Warm With The Raw!

Raw Pineapple, Chili, Cilantro, Lime and Ginger soup

This is a really great soup for dinner parties or when you are looking for something special. Additionally, the ingredients are great for digestion and detoxification.

In a blender, place serrano chilies that have been de-seeded, fresh ginger, fresh garlic, dried cumin, fresh cilantro, salt, and lime juice, blend well. Add the chopped fruit from a whole fresh pineapple, water and blend until smooth and soup is warm from the high-speed blender. Sprinkle lightly with cumin seeds and let sit in refrigerator overnight.

- 2 Serrano chilies
- 1 tablespoon chopped fresh ginger
- 2 teaspoons dried cumin
- 1/4 cup cilantro
- 2 or 3 limes
- 1 large fresh pineapple
- Sea salt to taste
- 1 teaspoon dried cumin

"Great for digestion and detoxification..."

Soups & Salads

Cure For The Garden: Featuring The Methionine Restriction Protocol   Copyright 2019. DocRhi.com

Eat The Warm With The Raw!

Soups & Salads

Crockpot Mexican Jackfruit Chili

- 2 cans green jackfruit, water drained off, wrung dry in cloth and mashed with a fork
- 1 large can of diced tomatoes
- 1 large can of chopped green chilies
- 1 small can of tomato paste or 1/2 cup enchilada sauce
- 1 large can of black beans
- 1 large can of pinto beans
- 1 can of slice mushrooms
- 1 deseeded and diced jalapeno pepper
- 1 onion, diced
- 1 bell pepper, diced
- 1 tablespoon ground dried shitake powder
- 1 teaspoon chili powder
- 2 tablespoons red wine vinegar
- 1 teaspoon each cumin and oregano
- Pinch of ground, dried stevia leaves

Place all ingredients, except lime, into slow cooker. Cook on high for 1-2 hours.

Tips for cooking with tofu and jack-fruit:

- Wring out jackfruit and extra-firm tofu in a cheese-cloth or thin kitchen towel by placing it in a towel and turning the ends of the towel in opposite directions just like wringing out laundry. Getting rid of the water helps give the tofu and jackfruit a firmer consistency.

Serve with a slice of lime to squeeze into bowl.

If you want to make 2 different chilis, swap out the jackfruit for refried beans.

Cure For The Garden: Featuring The Methionine Restriction Protocol   Copyright 2019. DocRhi.com

Eat The Warm With The Raw!

Soups & Salads

Miso Soup

Boil water in a large saucepan. Add chopped green onions, cubed tofu if you want it. Add Nori seaweed torn into strips. Add tamari sauce, white pepper, and ground ginger. Remove from heat and add miso. Stir until miso dissolves. Serve hot with stir-fried veggies or sushi. All spices can be altered for your taste buds.

- 4 cups water
- 3 green onions
- 1 cup of tofu
- 3 sheets of Nori seaweed torn in strips
- 1/2 teaspoon white pepper, ground
- 1/2 teaspoon ginger, ground
- 1 tablespoon tamari sauce or coconut aminos
- 2 1/2 tablespoons miso paste (It is important to make sure this paste does not have MSG and is non genetically engineered when you buy it!)
- 1 cup torn or chopped nettle leaves (optional)
- 1 clove chopped fresh garlic (optional)

"Seaweed is very important for the vegan diet as it contains Vitamin B12..."

Cooking with seaweed is very important for vegans as it contains Vitamin B12 as well as minerals such as iodine. Check out local Asian markets for a wide variety of seaweed and try out the different types to figure out the different flavors and textures.

Cure For The Garden: Featuring The Methionine Restriction Protocol   Copyright 2019. DocRhi.com

Eat The Warm With The Raw!

Soups & Salads

Black Bean Soup

Rinse and soak beans overnight. Rinse again and add 3 times the water to the amount of beans. Add all of the ingredients, except the oil and cook in a pressure cooker or on medium low on the stovetop until beans are soft and thick, about an hour in the

- 1 bag of black beans
- 1 onion
- 1 green bell pepper, chopped
- 1/4 cup cilantro
- 6 cloves of garlic
- 2 tablespoons of olive oil
- 2 tablespoons of balsamic vinegar
- 1 tablespoon of Dijon mustard (sugar free)
- 2 bay leaves
- 2 teaspoons cumin
- 2 teaspoons oregano
- 1/2 teaspoon cayenne
- 1/2 teaspoon black pepper
- A dash of sea salt to taste

Money saving tips for cooking with beans. Try to use one pot of beans for multiple uses. For example to make:

- Chili– add Tofu Burger patty crumbles or canned green jackfruit

- Burgers– drain water and pulse 2 cups bean soup in food processor with 1 tablespoon each of psyllium husk and flaxseed and 1/2 cup almond, yam, or plantain flour. Continue pulsing until a thick dough is formed. Mold into patties with hands and grill or dehydrate.

- Goulash– add a bag of lentil pasta, diced tomatoes and Italian spices (See spice section)

pressure cooker. Add olive oil and serve with fresh cilantro. Or, top with vinegar and chopped onion.

Cure For The Garden: Featuring The Methionine Restriction Protocol   Copyright 2019. DocRhi.com

Eat The Warm With The Raw!

Soups & Salads

Potato, Cauliflower, Pea And Onion Stew

Purée garlic, tomato and ginger.

Heat a skillet over medium heat. Add 2 tablespoons of water, pureed garlic mixture, onion, and turmeric. Heat a few minutes, stirring occasionally.

Add unpeeled, well scrubbed, chopped potatoes and 2 more tablespoons of water. Stir, cover and steam for about 3-5 minutes. Add cauliflower, tomato deseeded green chili, coriander, cumin, cinnamon, sea salt and paprika. Mix well, add 3 more tablespoons of water and cook 5 minutes. Add frozen peas and continue cooking until all vegetables are tender. Remove from heat and drizzle with virgin olive oil and top with chopped cilantro, zaatar or sumac (optional).

Serve hot over a bed of arugula or spinach greens with a side of hummus or baba ghanoush.

- 1 small chopped onion
- 1 cup of chopped cauliflower
- 1 small, deseeded chopped green chili
- 1 small chopped tomato
- 7 tablespoons water
- 2 tablespoons garlic
- 2 tablespoons ginger
- 1 1/2 teaspoon turmeric
- 1 1/2 teaspoon of coriander
- 1 teaspoon cumin
- 1 teaspoon cinnamon
- 1 teaspoon sea salt

Cure For The Garden: Featuring The Methionine Restriction Protocol

Baked Goods

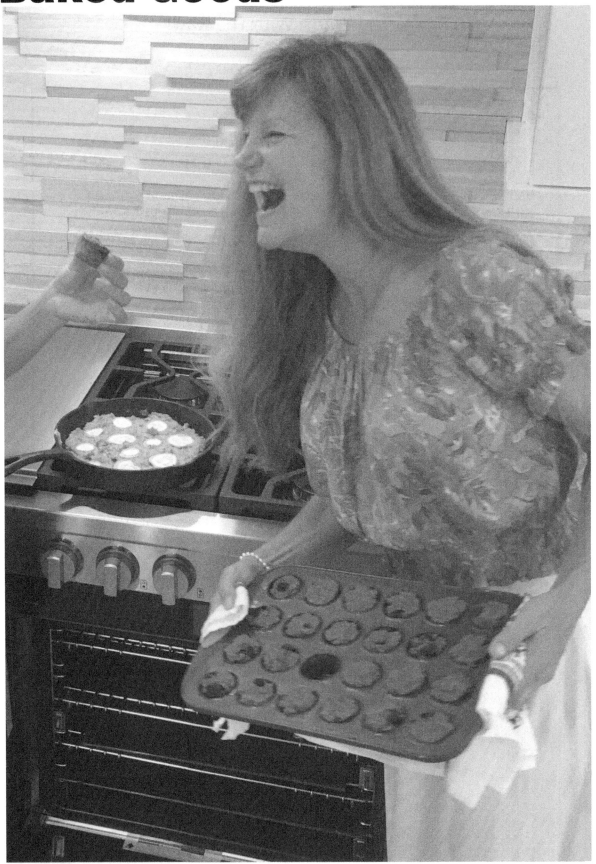

Cure For The Garden: Featuring The Methionine Restriction Protocol

Blow Anyone Away With Your Healthy Baking!

Sweet Potato Bread

Make your agua faba first by whisking the water from a can of garbanzo beans on high for 9 minutes or until it is firm enough to hold peaks when you lift a spoonful from it. Place cooked sweet potato into a food processor and blend until completely smooth. In a bowl, mix all dry ingredients, then mix in all wet ingredients. Fold in agua faba. Pour into an oiled and floured loaf pan and bake at 300F for 1– 1 1/2 hours until golden brown. Allow to cool completely before cutting.

- 1 1/2 cups flour (yam, potato, chick pea, lentil, coconut, or almond)

- 2 heaping tablespoons flax meal

- 2 heaping tablespoons psyllium husks

- 1 cup cooked sweet potato (or yam, pumpkin, potato, plantain or zucchini)

- 1 can agua faba (whisked water from a can of garbanzo beans)

- 1 teaspoon sea salt

- 1 teaspoon caraway (or rosemary, thyme, cinnamon & turmeric)

- 1 1/2 teaspoons aluminum-free baking powder

- 2 tablespoons sparkling water

- 1 tablespoon white vinegar

- 1 tablespoon agave or 1/2 teaspoon stevia

Cure For The Garden: Featuring The Methionine Restriction Protocol   Copyright 2019. DocRhi.com

Blow Anyone Away With Your Healthy Baking!

Banana and Walnut Muffins

Make your agua faba first by whisking the water from a can of garbanzo beans on high for 9 minutes or until it is firm enough to hold peaks when you lift a spoon out of it. In another bowl mash bananas and add all wet ingredients, except agua faba. In another bowl, mix all dry ingredients, mix thoroughly with wet ingredients, then fold in agua faba. Add walnuts or raisins, if desired.

- 2 bananas
- 2 cup almond flour
- 1 cup chickpea flour
- 1 teaspoon each of aluminum free baking powder and soda
- 1 teaspoon salt
- 1/2 teaspoon nutmeg
- 2 teaspoons cinnamon
- 1 tablespoon each flax meal and psyllium husk
- 2 bananas
- 1 1/2 teaspoons vanilla
- 3 tablespoons agave
- 12 drops liquid stevia
- 1 tablespoon white vinegar
- 2 tablespoons sparkling water
- 1/4 cup agua faba
- 1/4 cup each raisins and/ or chopped walnuts (optional)

Oil and flour a muffin pan and bake at 300F for 25-40 minutes depending upon the size of the muffins, or until an inserted toothpick comes out clean.

You can change this recipe up by substituting any nut or seed for the walnuts. You can also substitute cooked or apples, mangos, squash, pumpkin, carrots, or zucchini for the banana and substitute any dried fruit such as unsweetened cherries for the raisins!

Cure For The Garden: Featuring The Methionine Restriction Protocol   Copyright 2019. DocRhi.com

Blow Anyone Away With Your Healthy Baking!

Sprouted Lentil Flatbreads

Place lentils, flax, psyllium, sea salt and spices into food processor and mix until smooth. Stirring as needed. If too dry add water a teaspoon at a time until a dough like consistency. Roll into balls and flatten by hand. Bake in toaster oven until golden, in conventional oven at 350 F for 10 minutes and turn. Bake until golden or place into dehydrator and dry until crisp.

- 2 cups sprouted lentils, well drained
- 2 tablespoons flax meal
- 2 tablespoons psyllium husk
- Yam or almond flour as needed depending on the wetness of the lentils
- 1 teaspoon sea salt
- 1 teaspoon each of basil, fennel and rosemary (optional)
- Water as needed

"Repurpose your flatbreads into breakfast pizzas..."

To repurpose your flatbreads into breakfast pizzas: Top flat breads with choice of sauce (marinara, pesto or spinach artichoke dip and choice of vegetables like mushrooms, peppers, broccoli, olives, onions or any other. Add Italian spices and optional vegan parmesan or vegan cheese shreds. Place into toaster , or conventional oven at 400F until hot and vegan cheese has melted.

Baked Goods

Blow Anyone Away With Your Healthy Baking!

Quick Flatbread

Combine flour, psyllium husk, flax, cumin seeds, pepper, and salt and mix well. Add warm water as need to make smooth and pliable dough. Set aside for 10 minutes to allow mixture to bind.

- 1 cup chickpea flour
- 1/4 cup flax meal
- 1/8 cup of psyllium husk
- teaspoon salt or to taste
- 1/2 teaspoon cumin or rosemary seeds
- 1/8 teaspoon of red pepper flakes (optional)
- 1/3 cup water lukewarm use as needed
- 1/4 cup flour need for rolling the flat breads

Divide the dough in 6 equal parts.
Press both sides of a dough piece onto dry flour to make them easier to roll.

Roll them into six inch flat circles of even thickness throughout. While rolling, if your dough starts to stick to your rolling pin or rolling surface, you can sprinkle more flour as needed.

Place each piece on cookie sheet and let sit a few minutes prior to baking.

Bake in preheated oven set at 350F until light brown, about 25 minutes depending upon thickness. Then flip and bake a few more minutes.

Cure For The Garden: Featuring The Methionine Restriction Protocol

Copyright 2019. DocRhi.com

Blow Anyone Away With Your Healthy Baking!

Baked Goods

Pumpkin Kombucha Bread

This bread is a more traditional quick bread. You can slice it and use it as a normal bread. It slices really thin and can have an almost pumpernickel like taste and consistency, just be sure to let it cool completely before cutting. Don't worry! Any alcohol is cooked away and makes the bread lighter. Preheat oven to 300°F.

- 1 cup bean flour
- 1 cup almond or yam flour
- 1/8 cup each psyllium husk and flax meal
- 1 tablespoon white vinegar
- 1 teaspoon each aluminum free baking powder and soda
- 1 teaspoon sea salt
- 2 tablespoons raw agave nectar, or 1 cup pureed raisins or dates
- 1 teaspoon cinnamon
- 1/4 teaspoon each of nutmeg, ginger, cloves, allspice
- 1 cup kombucha or beer, your choice (we use ginger kombucha)
- 2 tablespoons tahini
- 1 can pumpkin or yam (or try savory potato with rosemary, thyme and olives instead of agave and the other spices)

"Remember, limiting to one slice per day keeps methionine levels low."

In a medium bowl combine all ingredients until flour is completely incorporated. Pour batter into a well oiled round cake or loaf pan and bake for 45-60 minutes, insert a knife in the middle of the loaf, when it comes out clean, it is done. Let cool completely!!! It is still cooking even through you have pulled it out of the oven.

Cure For The Garden: Featuring The Methionine Restriction Protocol   Copyright 2019. DocRhi.com

Blow Anyone Away With Your Healthy Baking!

Baked Goods

Gluten Free Bruschetta

Mix wet and dry ingredients separately before combining. Flatten by hand onto a non-stick or oiled and floured cookie sheet.

Bake immediately at 350F degrees for 25-30 minutes, until the top is golden.

Cut into rectangles and top with pesto, or marinara and veggies! Makes a meal for 2-3 or appetizers for 6-8. cook until golden.

Tip for switching any recipe to grain free!

Substitute flours for a blend of 3 parts yam, banana, or bean flour and 1 part nut flour. Use 1-2 tablespoons of psyllium husk and flax seed with very cold sparkling water instead of milk or regular water

- 1 1/2 cups chickpea, yam, banana, plantain or bean flour

- 1 cup nut or seed flour

- 1 teaspoon each baking soda and powder

- 1 tablespoon white vinegar

- 1 teaspoon sea salt

- 1 tablespoon each psyllium husk and flax meal

- 3/4–1 cup sparkling water

Blow Anyone Away With Your Healthy Baking!

Baked Goods

Sunflower Seed Tortillas

Food process sunflower seeds in an individual cup on high until they become a course flour-like consistency.

Add avocado and sunflower seeds to a regular food processor and process on high to blend.

Add psyllium husk, milled flax seed, almond flour, sea salt and food process on high to blend.

Add 3 tablespoons water and food process on high stopping and stirring occasionally until mix clumps slightly. Add 1-2 more tablespoons water as needed until mixture clumps slightly and sticks together when you squeeze it.

- 1/4 cup shelled raw sunflower seeds
- 2 medium or 1 large avocado
- 1/4 cup psyllium husk
- 2 tablespoons milled flax seed
- 1 cup almond or yam flour
- 1 teaspoon sea salt
- 3-5 tablespoons water

Allow dough to sit for 30 mins. Take 1 heaping tablespoon of dough and roll and squeeze back and forth between hands 12 times before placing on a tortilla press or hand flattening. Place flattened tortilla in toaster oven or baking sheet and bake on 325F for 4-8 minutes or until golden brown.

Makes 12 tortillas!

Cure For The Garden: Featuring The Methionine Restriction Protocol   Copyright 2019. DocRhi.com

Desserts

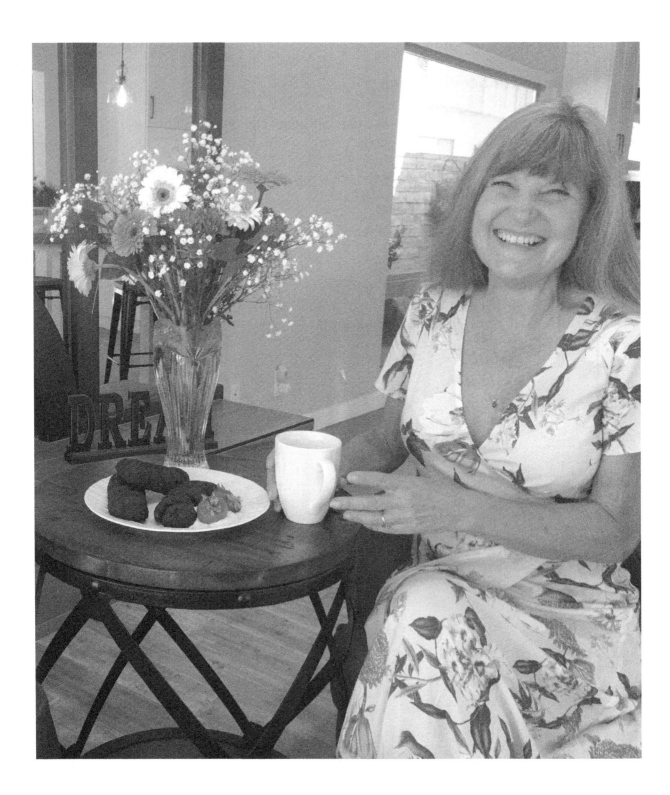

Cure For The Garden: Featuring The Methionine Restriction Protocol

Desserts So Healthy You Can Eat Them For Breakfast!

Gluten-free and Nut-free Pie Crust

- 1 1/2 cups yam or plantain flour
- 1 cup tahini
- 1/2 cup raw agave
- 1 teaspoon sea salt

Mix all the ingredients together and press into the bottom of a glass pan. Bake in over at 425F degrees for 20 minutes or until golden brown.

Cure For The Garden: Featuring The Methionine Restriction Protocol   Copyright 2019. DocRhi.com

Desserts So Healthy You Can Eat Them For Breakfast!

Desserts

Crust:

- 1 1/2 cup organic nuts and seeds
- 3/4 cup unsweetened dried coconut flakes
- 10 pitted dates or 1/2 cup raisins
- 1 teaspoon coconut oil
- Sea salt to taste

Raw Chocolate Avocado Fruit Tort Crust

Chop dates and other dried fruit in a food processor until creamy. Add all other ingredients to food processor and process until crumbly. Press the mixture into a tart pan or pie tin and gently press into the base and sides evenly, using slightly moistened fingertips.

Filling:

- 1-2 ripe avocados
- 1/2 cup - 2/3 cup raw cacao powder
- 1/8 cup frozen berries and cherries, drained of liquid
- 20 pitted dates
- 1/8 cup raisins
- 1 tablespoon agave syrup or stevia to taste
- Sea salt to taste

Chocolate Avocado Fruit Tort Filling

Place dates, raisins, and berries into food processor and blend well. Add avocados and cacao powder and mix until smooth. Add berries/cherries and pulse until mixture is creamy. Fold into crust in tart pan/ pie tin. Place in refrigerator for 1 hour prior to serving.

Cure For The Garden: Featuring The Methionine Restriction Protocol   Copyright 2019. DocRhi.com

Desserts So Healthy You Can Eat Them For Breakfast!

Compost Brownies

"Waste not, want not!" This is one of our favorite ways to stretch our food out to the maximum use.

Place juicing shreds into food processor and blend well. Add all remaining ingredients into food processor and blend until smooth. Roll dough into balls and flatten. Place on dehydrator rack and dry until chewy and warm. Serve with a cup of tea for breakfast or as dessert.

If you don't have a dehydrator, you can use a conventional oven at the lowest heat setting for 3 hours or until you can pull a clean knife out of the brownies.

- 1 cup juicing shreds
- 1 cup nuts or sprouted azuki beans
- 1 cup of raisins
- 2 tablespoons unsweetened cocoa
- 1 teaspoon sea salt
- 1 teaspoon vanilla
- stevia and agave to taste (We use 1 teaspoon of ground, dried stevia leaves)
- 1/2 cup unsweetened dried cherries or goji berries

Desserts So Healthy You Can Eat Them For Breakfast!

PB & J Brownies

Blend all wet ingredients, except sparkling water and agua faba, and mix well. In a separate bowl mix all dry ingredients. Combine wet and dry and mix thoroughly before mixing in sparkling water then folding in agua faba. If you use dryer flours such as yam flour you may add more water, stirring continuously, until batter is a pourable consistency. Pour into oiled and floured mini-bread pans or muffin pan and bake at 300F for 45 minutes then turn oven off and allow to stay in warm over for 30 more minutes.

- 1/2 cup almond butter

- 1/2 cup all fruit (fruit juice sweetened jelly without added sugar)

- 3/4 cup almond flour

- 3/4 cup chickpea/ garbanzo flour

- 4 tablespoons unsweetened cocoa

- 1 teaspoon sea salt

- 1 teaspoon vanilla

- stevia and agave to taste (We use 1 teaspoon of ground, dried stevia leaves and 2 tablespoons agave)

- 1 teaspoon each baking soda and powder

- 1 tablespoon vinegar

- 1/4 to 1/2 cup cold sparkling water

- 1 can agua faba (water from a can of garbanzo beans, whisked on high for 9 minutes or until it holds firm peaks)

Cure For The Garden: Featuring The Methionine Restriction Protocol   Copyright 2019. DocRhi.com

Desserts So Healthy You Can Eat Them For Breakfast!

Chocolate Cherry Covered Pears

These chocolate cherry covered pears are the fastest gourmet dessert we've ever made! For a party, cut up your pears and stick a toothpick in them for dipping, or serve smothered.

In a saucepan bring coconut milk, cacao, and jelly just to a simmer as you stir out any clumps with a fork. As soon as the mixture begins to boil, turn of the fire and add the stevia packets. Taste and add more if desired. Allow the mixture to cool for a minute as you cut the pears. Drizzle the chocolate over the pears or in a bowl for dipping!

Serves 4-6.

- 1/4 cup coconut milk
- 3 heaping tablespoons cocoa powder
- 2 heaping tablespoons cherry all fruit (fruit sweetened) or raspberry all fruit
- 2 sugar equivalent teaspoons stevia (2 packets)
- 3 green pears

When it comes to Stevia:

Most people think they do not like the taste of Stevia and that is because they have only ever tried the processed versions with additives like mannose and dextrose (other sugars). It is very important to use ground dried stevia leaf which you can order from many herb companies. You can also grow stevia and dry the leaves yourself. The flavor is completely different than the processed versions and doesn't have that strange aftertaste that the packets have so throw those out and get real!

Desserts So Healthy You Can Eat Them For Breakfast!

Tapioca Pudding

Tapioca pudding cups make a delicious dessert, are super easy, fast and you can easily swap fruit and add nuts for personalized favorites!

Add small pearl tapioca and water to a saucepan and soak overnight. Do not drain after soaking.

Add the nut/ seed milk and sea salt and cook over medium heat, stirring occasionally, until mixture comes to a gentle boil. Simmer uncovered over very low heat for 10 to 15 minutes, stirring occasionally, until mixture is thick. Remove from heat and cool for 15 minutes before stirring in pure maple syrup, stevia and vanilla extract. Either serve warm, or transfer to a sealable container and refrigerate until chilled.

Lastly, add the sliced bananas or other fruit of choice and enjoy!

Serves 3-4.

- 1/3 cup small pearl tapioca
- 3/4 cup water
- 1 cup nut or seed milk
- 2 tablespoons pure maple syrup
- Stevia to taste (We use 10 drops)
- pinch sea salt
- 1 teaspoon pure vanilla extract
- 1 cup fruit of choice (Such as sliced banana, fresh blueberries, chopped mango or kiwi)

Cure For The Garden: Featuring The Methionine Restriction Protocol   Copyright 2019. DocRhi.com

Drinking Your Meals!

Drinks

According to Oriental Medicine cold, frozen, raw, icy foods & drinks will eventually cause constitutional problems such as hypothyroidism, pain, fatigue, sinus infections and obesity. The reason for this is that each time you consume something cold or completely raw it takes more digestive energy to break it down. Smoothies should be warmed up with water from your teapot if you are using frozen fruit so they are served room temperature and they should have vegetables as well as fruit! Add warming herbs such as cinnamon or ginger to counter the cold/ raw quality. You can enjoy them, even in the winter when it is cool out! If you add a little agave and stevia (and we like a couple of tablespoons full of unsweetened baking cocoa) to any smoothie with berries and any green vegetables with warm water, you can change up the flavors. Smoothies are also a great way to use your produce before it goes bad, and get lots of plant nutrients!

- 2 cups spinach

- 1 cup coconut water

- About 1/4 teaspoon of fresh ginger (You don't need to grind it since the blender will do this for you. Cut a piece of ginger about the size of the end of your pinky finger.)

- The juice of 1 lemon

- 1 green pear cored

- 1 green apple cored

Drink Your Greens Smoothie

Blend the pear, apple, lemon juice, coconut water, ginger, and as much spinach as will fit in the blender. Blend on high. Add more coconut water as needed to blend up solids. When blended add the rest of the spinach or use foraged greens if you have them available such as stinging nettles, chickweed, or purslane. You can check out the book "Forage and Feed Your Family" for more great info on foraging for nutrient packed wild foods.

"Check out the book "Forage and Feed Your Family" for more great info on foraging for nutrient packed wild foods..."

Cure For The Garden: Featuring The Methionine Restriction Protocol   Copyright 2019. DocRhi.com

Drinking Your Meals!

Chai Tea

This is an excellent tea to have made for parties instead of coffee. You can make it as sweet and milky as you'd like and even save the rest in the refrigerator to drink cold. Heat all ingredients except vanilla and nut milk in a covered non-metallic pan for 10 minutes. Add nut/seed milk and simmer on low for another 10 minutes. Sprinkle with nutmeg and a few drops of vanilla extract; sweeten with stevia and raw agave.

- About 1" of fresh ginger root, finely grated

- 6 black peppercorns

- 2 cinnamon sticks

- 5 cloves

- 12 cardamom seeds

- 1/2 teaspoon ground nutmeg

- 1-2 teaspoons vanilla

- 2 1/2 cups water

- 1/2 cup nut or tahini milk (Optionally make your own by blending 2 tablespoons creamy nut butter or tahini with 1 cup water)

"An excellent tea to have made for parties instead of coffee..."

Cure For The Garden: Featuring The Methionine Restriction Protocol   Copyright 2019. DocRhi.com

Methionine Restriction Calculations

For those that want to do the precise measurements by hand, here are the calculations to figure out exactly how much methionine you can eat for an 80% restriction.

If you want to find the amount of methionine you can eat with an 80% restriction just place your perfect weight in the formula below. No weighing is needed because you use your ideal weight, not your current weight!

1. Convert your perfect weight in pounds (lbs.) to kilograms

To find this, multiply your perfect weight in lbs. by 0.454 = Your perfect weight in kilograms. We'll call this number "X".

2. Find how many milligrams of methionine you can eat each day.

To do this, multiply "X" by .038mg/kg. = the amount of methionine in milligrams you can eat each day. We'll call this number "M."

3. Then divide that number by 1000 to convert milligrams to grams of methionine you can eat each day.

.038mg/kg a day of methionine is an 80% restriction of the standard recommended daily value. As a reminder, this is a research-based strict methionine restriction recommendation. **Each person has individual health goals and should work with a Certified Methionine Restriction Protocol Coach and primary care physician who can carefully monitor and adjust daily methionine recommendations, supplements and pharmaceutical prescriptions as needed.**

Methionine Restriction Calculations

More examples:

Let's say you are a woman that dreams of weighing 120 lbs.

First we need to convert the ideal weight in pounds to kilograms

(120 lbs. to kilograms is 1 lb. to .454 kg./lbs.)

120lb*0.454kg/lb.= 54.4kg of body weight.

Then we want to know how many grams of methionine she should eat each day for the ideal weight in kilograms. 80% of the recommended methionine requirement is 3.8g per kilogram of body weight.

(54.4 kg*3.8mg methionine for each kilogram of body weight=206mg methionine/day/1000 to convert from mg to g= 0.206g methionine/day)

So, she can have .206g of methionine each day.

A man wanting to weigh 160 lbs. would use this formula:

160lb*0.454kg/lb.= 72.6kg

72.6kg*3.8mg/kg= 276mg or

0.276g methionine/day

The overall idea is to prepare dishes that contain mostly low methionine foods with a little or no high methionine foods added. Once you have reached your methionine allowance for the day, eat from the .001 or .002 methionine foods until you are satisfied.

Next, we will discuss the calculations to find the amount of any one particular food you can eat in a day, depending upon its methionine content. Of course, you don't want to eat all of your methionine in one food so be sure to eat only about 1/3 or 1/4 of the food amount allowed and add methionine from other foods to ensure a rainbow of phytochemicals, anti oxidants and nutrients every day.

Methionine Restriction Calculations

If we take the example of the man who wants to weigh 160 lbs. he is allowed 0.276g of methionine/day.

Dry roasted almonds contain 0.155g methionine per 100g of almonds. (On the chart we have listed 100g in cups so that it is easier to visualize for those of us using cup measurements).

You divide 0.276g/0.155g=1.78g of methionine

Multiply 1.78 by the amount of cups of the almonds, which is 0.7 cups.

1.78 * 0.7 cups = 1.25 or 1 1/4 cups of almonds that you can eat per day.

However, you don't want to eat all of your methionine allowance in just 1 food or in just 1 meal.

So, divide that amount, 1 1/4 cup by 1/4 and you can eat a little more than 1/4 cup of almonds for the day and still leave 3/4 of your methionine allowance for the rest of your foods. You can see that if you want to carry almonds as a snack you could easily do so and mix in produce like dried cherries and raisins to add bulk without adding a lot of methionine.

To find the amount of methionine in the 1/4 cup of almonds, divide the methionine amount in the food list for almonds by four (since you are only eating about 1/4 the amount listed). 0.155g/4 gives you the total grams of methionine you have eaten in that 1/4 cup of almonds.

0.155/4=.038g of methionine in 1/4 cup almonds.

Subtract the amount of methionine found in 1/4 cup of almonds from the total amount of methionine per day you can have for your ideal weight.

0.276g - 0.038g= 0.238g left for the rest of the day.

You can see that this is just addition, subtraction, multiplication and division. Still, it can get tedious. Try to simply eat fruits and vegetables and leave the beans, seeds, and nuts for sauces and baked goods with lots of produce mixed in. For example, the pumpkin kombucha bread recipe uses produce mixed in with the nut or bean flour to reduce the total methionine in the loaf of bread.

Cure For The Garden: Featuring The Methionine Restriction Protocol

Instructions For Using The Food Chart

Here are some general ways you can use the food chart without having to calculate each meal:

If the grams of methionine contained in 100 grams of the food is 0.01 or less, eat all you want!

If the grams of methionine contained in 100 grams of the food is 0.01 to 0.03, eat up to twice the cup amount listed, or 200 grams of the food.

If the grams of methionine contained in 100 grams of the food is 0.03 to 0.05, eat less than or up to the amount listed on the food chart, or 100 grams of the food.

If the grams of methionine contained in 100 grams of the food is 0.05 to 0.1, eat only up to 1/2 the cup amount listed or 50 grams of the food.

If the grams of methionine contained in the 100 grams of the food is 0.1 to 0.2, eat only up to 1/10 the cup amount listed or 10 grams of the food.

If the grams of methionine contained in the 100 grams of the food is 2 to 0.5 eat only 1/20 of the cup amount listed or 5 grams of the food.

If the grams of methionine contained in the 100 grams of the food is over 0.5, chose to eat only trace amounts for flavor in recipes and then only a small amount, like one slice of bread, etc.

This adds to .06 + .05 +.05 + 0.02 + .025 + trace say 0.05= 0.255 which is great for the 160 lb. man but a little high for the 120 lb. woman.

Remember you only restrict the high methionine foods. The low methionine foods towards the top of the list are all you can eat!

We know you are thinking, this is seriously hard!

This is easier than it seems!

Cure For The Garden: Featuring The Methionine Restriction Protocol   Copyright 2019. DocRhi.com

Low Methionine Food Chart (Listed Lowest To Highest)

Salt, table	0	
Vinegar, cider	0	
Dandelion greens	0	
Psyllium husk	0	
Cilantro	0	
Tea black	0	
Coffee brewed grounds	0	
Artichoke globe	0	
Quince	0	
Honey	0	
Prickly pear tuna	0	
Wine	0	
Apples, raw, golden delicious, with skin	0.001	1/2 medium apple
Apples, raw, red delicious, with skin	0.001	1/2 medium apple
Apples, raw, with skin	0.001	1/2 medium apple
Apples, raw, without skin	0.001	1/2 medium apple
Chayote, fruit, cooked, boiled, drained, with salt	0.001	.76 of a cup 1"pieces
Chayote, fruit, cooked, boiled, drained, without salt	0.001	.76 of a cup 1"pieces
Chayote, fruit, raw	0.001	.76 of a cup 1"pieces
Grape juice, canned or bottled, unsweetened, with added ascorbic acid and calcium	0.001	.40 of cup
Grape juice, canned or bottled, unsweetened, without added ascorbic acid	0.001	.40 of cup
Strawberries, canned, heavy syrup pack, solids and liquids	0.001	.69 cup
Strawberries, frozen, sweetened, sliced	0.001	3/5 cup
Strawberries, frozen, sweetened, whole	0.001	.69 cup
Strawberries, frozen, unsweetened	0.001	.69 cup
Apples, canned, sweetened, sliced, drained, heated	0.002	.39 cup
Apples, canned, sweetened, sliced, drained, unheated	0.002	.39 cup
Apples, dried, sulfured, stewed, without added sugar	0.002	.39 cup
Applesauce, canned, unsweetened, with added ascorbic acid	0.002	.39 cup
Applesauce, canned, unsweetened, without added ascorbic acid	0.002	.39 cup
Applesauce, canned, unsweetened, without added ascorbic acid	0.002	.39 cup
Guava sauce, cooked	0.002	.42 cup
Lime juice, raw	0.002	.41 cup
Limes, raw	0.002	2 1/4 cup
Noodles, Chinese, mung beans, dehydrated	0.002	.71 cup
Onions, raw	0.002	1 cup
Onions, yellow, sautéed	0.002	1 cup
Orange juice, chilled, includes from concentrate	0.002	.40 cup 2/5 cup
Orange juice, chilled, includes from concentrate, with added calcium	0.002	.40 cup 2/5 cup
Orange juice, chilled, includes from concentrate, with added calcium and vitamin D	0.002	.40 cup 2/5 cup
Orange juice, chilled, includes from concentrate, with added calcium and vitamins A, D, E	0.002	.40 cup
Papayas, raw	0.002	.43 cups mashed
Pears, canned, extra heavy syrup pack, solids and liquids	0.002	.71 cup sliced
Pears, canned, heavy syrup pack, solids and liquids	0.002	.71 cup sliced
Pears, canned, light syrup pack, solids and liquids	0.002	.71 cup sliced
Pears, canned, water pack, solids and liquids	0.002	.71 cup sliced
Pears, canned, water pack, solids and liquids	0.002	.71 cup sliced

Cure For The Garden: Featuring The Methionine Restriction Protocol   Copyright 2019. DocRhi.com

Pears, raw, bartlett	0.002	1/2 medium
Pears, raw, bosc	0.002	1/2 medium
Pears, raw, red anjou	0.002	1/2 medium
Strawberries, raw	0.002	.69 cup
Tangerine juice, canned, sweetened	0.002	.40 cup
Tangerine juice, raw	0.002	.40 cup
Tangerines, (mandarin oranges), raw	0.002	.40 cup 2/5 cup
Tapioca	0.002	
Molasses	0.002	
Apples, dehydrated (low moisture), sulfured, stewed	0.003	.36 cup
Apples, frozen, unsweetened, heated	0.003	.36 cup
Apples, frozen, unsweetened, unheated	0.003	.36 cup
Apples, raw, without skin, cooked, microwave	0.003	.36 cup
Apples, raw, without skin, cooked, microwave	0.003	.36 cup
Apples, raw, without skin, cooked, microwave	0.003	.36 cup
Apricots, canned, extra light syrup pack, with skin, solids and liquids	0.003	.65 cup halves
Apricots, canned, juice pack, with skin, solids and liquids	0.003	.65 cup halves
Apricots, canned, light syrup pack, with skin, solids and liquids	0.003	.65 cup halves
Apricots, canned, water pack, without skin, solids and liquids	0.003	.65 cup halves
Cranberries, raw	0.003	.91 cup chopped
Figs, canned, light syrup pack, solids and liquids	0.003	.67 cup
Figs, canned, water pack, solids and liquids	0.003	.67 cup
Orange juice, canned, unsweetened	0.003	.40 cup 2/5 cup
Orange juice, raw	0.003	.40 cup 2/5 cup
Pears, raw, green anjou	0.003	.71 cup sliced 1/2 medium
Pickles, cucumber, sour	0.003	.65 cup apr. 2/3 cup
Pickles, cucumber, sour, low sodium	0.003	.65 cup apr. 2/3 cup
Plums, canned, purple, light syrup pack, solids and liquids	0.003	.40 cup 2/5 cup
Plums, canned, purple, water pack, solids and liquids	0.003	.40 cup 2/5 cup
Sapodilla, raw	0.003	.41 cups
Waxgourd, (chinese preserving melon), cooked, boiled, drained, with salt	0.003	.76 cup
Waxgourd, (chinese preserving melon), cooked, boiled, drained, without salt	0.003	.76 cup
Waxgourd, (chinese preserving melon), raw	0.003	.76 cup cubed
Apricots, canned, water pack, with skin, solids and liquids	0.004	.65 cup halves
Carrots, canned, no salt added, drained solids	0.004	.82 cup
Carrots, canned, regular pack, solids and liquids	0.004	.82 cup
Crabapples, raw	0.004	.91 cup sliced
Gourd, white-flowered (calabash), cooked, boiled, drained, with salt	0.004	.5 cup 1/2 cup 1" pieces
Gourd, white-flowered (calabash), cooked, boiled, drained, without salt	0.004	.5 cup 1/2 cup 1" pieces
Gourd, white-flowered (calabash), raw	0.004	.5 cup 1/2 cup 1" pieces
Guavas, strawberry, raw	0.004	.41 cup
Loquats, raw	0.004	6 & 1/4 loquats
Pears, canned, extra light syrup pack, solids and liquids	0.004	1/2 cup
Pears, canned, juice pack, solids and liquids	0.004	1/2 cup
Plums, canned, purple, juice pack, solids and liquids	0.004	.40 cup 2/5 cup
Noni	0.004	
Raspberry	0.004	
Apricots, dried, sulfured, stewed, without added sugar	0.005	.40 cup 2/5 cup
Celery, raw	0.005	5 & 3/4 stalks 5" long
Chicory, witloof, raw	0.005	1.1 cup

Cure For The Garden: Featuring The Methionine Restriction Protocol   Copyright 2019. DocRhi.com

171

Food		
Grapefruit, raw, pink and red, California and Arizona	0.005	.43 cup
Grapefruit, raw, pink and red, Florida	0.005	.43 cup
Grapefruit, sections, canned, light syrup pack, solids and liquids	0.005	.41 cup
Grapefruit, sections, canned, water pack, solids and liquids	0.005	.41 cup
Lettuce, iceberg (includes crisphead types), raw	0.005	1.39 cup shred, 12 leaves
Melons, honeydew, raw	0.005	.59 cup diced 3/5 cup
Peppers, sweet, red, frozen, chopped, boiled, drained, with salt	0.005	.67 cup
Peppers, sweet, red, frozen, chopped, boiled, drained, without salt	0.005	.67 cup
Persimmons, japanese, raw	0.005	3/5 medium fruit
Pickles, cucumber, dill or kosher dill	0.005	.65 cup sliced
Pickles, cucumber, dill, reduced sodium	0.005	.65 cup sliced
Tomato juice, canned, without salt added	0.005	.41 cup
Tomato products, canned, sauce, with onions, green peppers, and celery	0.005	1.66 cup
Apricots, raw	0.006	.65 cup
Blueberries, frozen, sweetened	0.006	.69 cup
Carrots, baby, raw	0.006	.82 cup strips or slices
Cucumber, with peel, raw	0.006	1 & 7/8 cup
Figs, raw	0.006	2/3 cup chopped
Grapefruit, raw, pink and red and white, all areas	0.006	.43 cup
Grapefruit, raw, white, Florida	0.006	.43 cup
Nectarines, raw	0.006	2/3 medium .70 cup sliced
Onions, frozen, chopped, cooked, boiled, drained, with salt	0.006	little less than 1/2 cup
Onions, frozen, chopped, cooked, boiled, drained, without salt	0.006	little less than 1/2 cup .48 cup
Onions, frozen, whole, cooked, boiled, drained, with salt	0.006	little less than 1/2 cup .48 cup
Onions, frozen, whole, cooked, boiled, drained, without salt	0.006	little less than 1/2 cup .48 cup
Pears, asian, raw	0.006	1/2 medium
Peppers, sweet, red, raw	0.006	.67 cup
Peppers, sweet, red, sauteed	0.006	.67 cup
Radishes, oriental, cooked, boiled, drained, with salt	0.006	.86 cup
Radishes, oriental, cooked, boiled, drained, without salt	0.006	.68 cup
Radishes, oriental, raw	0.006	.86 cup
Tomatoes, red, ripe, raw, year round average	0.006	3/4 med, 5 3/4 cherry, 1 2/3 roma
Vegetable juice cocktail, canned	0.006	.40 cup 2/5 cup
Vegetable juice cocktail, low sodium, canned	0.006	.40 cup 2/5 cup
Watermelon, raw	0.006	.66 cup diced 2/3 cup
Arrowroot flour	0.006	
Blueberries, frozen, unsweetened	0.007	.69 cup
Cabbage, chinese (pe-tsai), raw	0.007	1.32 cup shredded
Carrots, frozen, unprepared	0.007	.68 cup
Celery, cooked, boiled, drained, with salt	0.007	.67 cup diced
Celery, cooked, boiled, drained, without salt	0.007	.67 cup diced
Feijoa, raw	0.007	1/2 cup 1/2" chunks
Grapefruit, raw, pink and red, all areas	0.007	.43 cup
Grapefruit, raw, white, all areas	0.007	.43 cup
Grapefruit, sections, canned, juice pack, solids and liquids	0.007	.41 cup
Onions, canned, solids and liquids	0.007	.43 cup diced
Peppers, sweet, green, raw	0.007	.67 > 2/3 cup
Peppers, sweet, green, sauteed	0.007	.67 > 2/3 cup
Persimmons, native, raw	0.007	3/5 medium fruit
Soursop, raw	0.007	.44 cup pulp
Squash, winter, spaghetti, cooked, boiled, drained, or baked	0.007	.65 < 2/3 cup

Low Methionine Food List

Cure For The Garden: Featuring The Methionine Restriction Protocol   Copyright 2019. DocRhi.com

172

Squash, winter, spaghetti, raw	0.007	.65 < 2/3 cup
Sugar-apples, (sweetsop), raw	0.007	.40 cup pulp
Taro, cooked, with salt	0.007	.76 cup sliced
Taro, cooked, without salt	0.007	.76 cup sliced < 3/4
Tomato products, canned, sauce, spanish style	0.007	1 &2/3 cup
Tomato products, canned, sauce, spanish style	0.007	1 &2/3 cup
Yambean (jicama), raw	0.007	.77 cup
Bananas, raw	0.008	3/4 medium fruit .67 cup sliced
Grapefruit, raw, white, California	0.008	.43 cup 1/3 fruit
Mangos, raw	0.008	.61 cup 1 & 1/2 medium fruit
Plums, raw	0.008	.61 cup 1 & 1/2 medium fruit
Pumpkin, cooked, boiled, drained, with salt	0.008	.41 cup
Pumpkin, cooked, boiled, drained, without salt	0.008	.41 cup
Radicchio, raw	0.008	.40 cup
Squash, winter, acorn, cooked, boiled, mashed, with salt	0.008	.41 cup
Squash, winter, acorn, cooked, boiled, mashed, without salt	0.008	.42 cup
Tomato products, canned, sauce	0.008	.41 cup
Tomato sauce, canned, no salt added	0.008	.41 cup
Tomatoes, red, ripe, canned, packed in tomato juice	0.008	.42 cup
Tomatoes, red, ripe, canned, packed in tomato juice, no salt added	0.008	.42 cup
Tomatoes, red, ripe, canned, stewed	0.008	.41 cup
Tomatoes, yellow, raw	0.008	.72 cup chopped
Apples, dried, sulfured, uncooked	0.009	.63 cup
Beans, snap, green, canned, no salt added, solids and liquids	0.009	.65 cup
Beans, snap, green, canned, regular pack, solids and liquids	0.009	.65 cup
Beans, snap, yellow, canned, no salt added, solids and liquids	0.009	.65 cup
Beans, snap, yellow, canned, regular pack, solids and liquids	0.009	.65 cup
Beets, canned, no salt added, solids and liquids	0.009	.41 cup
Beets, canned, regular pack, solids and liquids	0.009	.44 cup
Beets, pickled, canned, solids and liquids	0.009	.44 cup
Burdock root, raw	0.009	.85 cup 1" pieces
Cabbage, chinese (pak-choi), cooked, boiled, drained, with salt	0.009	.84 cup
Cabbage, chinese (pak-choi), cooked, boiled, drained, without salt	0.009	.84 cup
Cabbage, chinese (pak-choi), raw	0.009	1.43 cup shredded
Cabbage, chinese (pe-tsai), cooked, boiled, drained, with salt	0.009	.84 cup
Cabbage, chinese (pe-tsai), cooked, boiled, drained, without salt	0.009	.84 cup
Eggplant, cooked, boiled, drained, with salt	0.009	1 cup 1" cubes
Eggplant, cooked, boiled, drained, without salt	0.009	1 cup 1" cubes
Grapes, red or green (European type, such as Thompson seedless), raw	0.009	.66 cup 20 fruits
Litchis, raw	0.009	.53 cup 10 fruits
Onions, sweet, raw	0.009	.48 cup
Oranges, raw, navels	0.009	.71 fruit .61 cup sectioned
Peppers, chili, green, canned	0.009	.72 cup
Pineapple, canned, light syrup pack, solids and liquids	0.009	.38 cup crushed sliced or chunks
Sauerkraut, canned, solids and liquids	0.009	.70 cup
Squash, summer, crookneck and straightneck, canned, drained, solid, without salt	0.009	.79 cup
Squash, summer, zucchini, includes skin, cooked, boiled, drained, with salt	0.009	.45 cup
Squash, summer, zucchini, includes skin, cooked, boiled, drained, without salt	0.009	.45 cup

Cure For The Garden: Featuring The Methionine Restriction Protocol   Copyright 2019. DocRhi.com

173

Tomato products, canned, puree, with salt added	0.009	.43 cup
Tomato products, canned, puree, without salt added	0.009	.43 cup
Tomatoes, red, ripe, cooked	0.009	.43 cup
Tomatoes, red, ripe, cooked, with salt	0.009	.43 cup
Turnips, cooked, boiled, drained, with salt	0.009	.43 cup mashed
Turnips, cooked, boiled, drained, without salt	0.009	.43 cup
Agave syrup raw	0.009	
Apricots, dehydrated (low-moisture), sulfured, stewed	0.01	.40 cup 2/5 cup
Beans, snap, canned, all styles, seasoned, solids and liquids	0.01	.42 cup
Beets, canned, drained solids	0.01	.44 cup
Beets, harvard, canned, solids and liquids	0.01	.44 cup
Blueberries, canned, heavy syrup, solids and liquids	0.01	.39 cup
Breadfruit, raw	0.01	.45 cup
Celtuce, raw	0.01	2.cups shredded
Cherries, sweet, raw	0.01	.72 cup with pits 12 cherries
Chicory greens, raw	0.01	3.45 cups
Leeks, (bulb and lower leaf-portion), cooked, boiled, drained, with salt	0.01	.96 cup
Leeks, (bulb and lower leaf-portion), cooked, boiled, drained, without salt	0.01	.96 cup
Orange juice, frozen concentrate, unsweetened, undiluted	0.01	.35 cup
Orange juice, frozen concentrate, unsweetened, undiluted, with added calcium	0.01	.35 cup
Peaches, canned, extra light syrup, solids and liquids	0.01	.40 cup
Peaches, yellow, raw	0.01	.77 cup
Peppers, hungarian, raw	0.01	.81 cup
Peppers, sweet, green, canned, solids and liquids	0.01	.71 cup
Peppers, sweet, red, canned, solids and liquids	0.01	.71 cup
Pickles, cucumber, sweet (includes bread and butter pickles)	0.01	.65 cup sliced 3 pickles
Plantains, cooked	0.01	.85 fried green 1/2 cup mashed .65 sliced
Radishes, raw	0.01	.86 cup sliced 50 small fruits
Radishes, white icicle, raw	0.01	1 cup sliced
Squash, winter, acorn, raw	0.01	.71 cup cubes
Tangerines, (mandarin oranges), canned, light syrup pack	0.01	.40 cup
Tomato products, canned, sauce, with onions	0.01	.41 cup
Tomatoes, green, raw	0.01	.56 cup 1.1 smal fruit
Tomatoes, orange, raw	0.01	.63 cup .90 fruit
Cassava, raw	0.011	.49 cup
Dill weed, fresh	0.011	11.24 cup
Eggplant, raw	0.011	1.22 cup
Onions, cooked, boiled, drained, with salt	0.011	.48 cup
Onions, cooked, boiled, drained, without salt	0.011	.48 cup
Peaches, canned, light syrup pack, solids and liquids	0.011	.40 cup
Peaches, canned, water pack, solids and liquids	0.011	.41 cup
Pears, dried, sulfured, stewed, without added sugar	0.011	.39 cup halves
Peas, edible-podded, frozen, unprepared	0.011	.69 cup
Peas, edible-podded, raw	0.011	1 cup
Peppers, hot chili, green, canned, pods, excluding seeds, solids and liquids	0.011	2.94 cup
Peppers, hot chili, red, canned, excluding seeds, solids and liquids	0.011	.74 cup
Peppers, sweet, green, cooked, boiled, drained, with salt	0.011	.74 cup
Peppers, sweet, green, cooked, boiled, drained, without salt	0.011	.74 cup chopped or strips

Low Methionine Food List

Cure For The Garden: Featuring The Methionine Restriction Protocol   Copyright 2019. DocRhi.com

Peppers, sweet, green, frozen, chopped, cooked, boiled, drained, with salt	0.011	.74 cup
Peppers, sweet, red, cooked, boiled, drained, with salt	0.011	.74 cup
Peppers, sweet, red, cooked, boiled, drained, without salt	0.011	.74 cup
Pineapple, canned, juice pack, solids and liquids	0.011	.40 crushed sliced chunks, 2.13 rings
Pineapple, canned, water pack, solids and liquids	0.011	.40 crushed sliced chunks, 2.13 rings
Pineapple, frozen, chunks, sweetened	0.011	.41 cup
Pumpkin, raw	0.011	.86 cup cubes
Squash, winter, all varieties, cooked, baked, with salt	0.011	.49 cup
Squash, winter, all varieties, cooked, baked, without salt	0.011	.49 cup
Squash, winter, butternut, cooked, baked, with salt	0.011	.49 cup
Squash, winter, butternut, cooked, baked, without salt	0.011	.48 cup cubes
Turnips, raw	0.011	.77 cup .82 medium
Rice wild (North American)	0.011	
Blueberries, raw	0.012	.68 cup
Burdock root, cooked, boiled, drained, with salt	0.012	.80 cup
Burdock root, cooked, boiled, drained, without salt	0.012	.80 cup
Cabbage, common (danish, domestic, and pointed types), freshly harvest, raw	0.012	1.43 cups
Cabbage, common (danish, domestic, and pointed types), stored, raw	0.012	1.43 cup .11 head
Cabbage, common, cooked, boiled, drained, with salt	0.012	.66 cup 2/3 head
Cabbage, cooked, boiled, drained, without salt	0.012	.66 cup
Cabbage, raw	0.012	1.43 cup
Cucumber, peeled, raw	0.012	.84 cup sliced
Melons, cantaloupe, raw	0.012	.63 cup .18 fruit medium
Olives, ripe, canned (small-extra large)	0.012	.75 cup
Olives, ripe, canned (small-extra large)	0.012	.75 cup
Peppers, jalapeno, canned, solids and liquids	0.012	.74 cups chopped
Peppers, sweet, yellow, raw	0.012	.67 cup
Persimmons, japanese, dried	0.012	.60 fruit
Pineapple, raw, all varieties	0.012	.61 cup .11 fruit
Pumpkin pie mix, canned	0.012	.37 cup
Pumpkin, canned, with salt	0.012	.41 cup
Pumpkin, canned, without salt	0.012	.41 cup
Squash, summer, crookneck and straightneck, frozen, unprepared	0.012	.77 cup sliced
Squash, winter, butternut, raw	0.012	.71 cup cubes
Apples, dehydrated (low moisture), sulfured, uncooked	0.013	1.67 cup
Beans, snap, green, canned, no salt added, drained solids	0.013	.65 cup
Beans, snap, green, canned, regular pack, drained solids	0.013	.65 cup
Carrots, canned, no salt added, solids and liquids	0.013	.41 cup
Carrots, frozen, cooked, boiled, drained, with salt	0.013	.68 cup
Carrots, frozen, cooked, boiled, drained, without salt	0.013	.68 cup
Escarole, cooked, boiled, drained, no salt added	0.013	.66 cup
Ginger root, raw	0.013	1 cup
Kohlrabi, raw	0.013	.74 cup
Longans, raw	0.013	30 fruit
Nuts, coconut water (liquid from coconuts)	0.013	.42 cup
Peas, edible-podded, boiled, drained, without salt	0.013	.63 cup
Peas, edible-podded, cooked, boiled, drained, with salt	0.013	.63 cup
Peppers, sweet, green, frozen, chopped, unprepared	0.013	.63 cup

Cure For The Garden: Featuring The Methionine Restriction Protocol

Low Methionine Food List

Peppers, sweet, red, frozen, chopped, unprepared	0.013	.63 cup
Pimento, canned	0.013	.52 cup
Squash, summer, all varieties, cooked, boiled, drained, with salt	0.013	.48 cup
Squash, summer, all varieties, cooked, boiled, drained, without salt	0.013	.48 cup
Squash, summer, crookneck and straightneck, cooked, boiled, drained, with salt	0.013	.48 cup
Squash, summer, crookneck and straightneck, cooked, boiled, drained, without salt	0.013	.48 cup
Tangerines, (mandarin oranges), canned, juice pack	0.013	.40 cup
Tomatoes, crushed, canned	0.013	.83 cup
Turnips, frozen, unprepared	0.013	.61 cup
Beans, snap, yellow, canned, no salt added, drained solids	0.014	.65 cup
Beans, snap, yellow, canned, regular pack, drained solids	0.014	.65 cup
Cabbage, red, cooked, boiled, drained, with salt	0.014	.67 cup
Cabbage, red, cooked, boiled, drained, without salt	0.014	.67 cup
Cabbage, red, raw	0.014	1.43 cup
Carrots, canned, regular pack, drained solids	0.014	.41 cup
Elderberries, raw	0.014	.69 cup
Endive, raw	0.014	2 cup
Kohlrabi, cooked, boiled, drained, with salt	0.014	.61 cup
Kohlrabi, cooked, boiled, drained, without salt	0.014	.84 cup
Lettuce, butterhead (includes boston and bibb types), raw	0.014	1.82 cup
Lotus root, cooked, boiled, drained, with salt	0.014	.84 cup
Lotus root, cooked, boiled, drained, without salt	0.014	.84 cup
Olives, ripe, canned (jumbo-super colossal)	0.014	.5 cup
Peas, edible-podded, frozen, cooked, boiled, drained, with salt	0.014	.63 cup
Peas, edible-podded, frozen, cooked, boiled, drained, without salt	0.014	.63 cup
Purslane, cooked, boiled, drained, with salt	0.014	.87 cup
Purslane, cooked, boiled, drained, without salt	0.014	.87 cup
Sesbania flower, cooked, steamed, with salt	0.014	.96 cup
Sesbania flower, cooked, steamed, without salt	0.014	.96 cup
Squash, summer, crookneck and straightneck, raw	0.014	.77 cup sliced
Squash, winter, acorn, cooked, baked, with salt	0.014	.49 cup
Squash, winter, acorn, cooked, baked, without salt	0.014	.49 cup
Tamarinds, raw	0.014	.83 cup pulp
Tomato products, canned, sauce, with mushrooms	0.014	.41 cup
Cassava root	0.014	
Apricots, dried, sulfured, uncooked	0.015	.40 cup 2/5 cup
Figs, dried, stewed	0.015	.39 cup
Lettuce, cos or romaine, raw	0.015	2.13 cup shredded .16 head
Mushrooms, maitake, raw	0.015	1.43 cup diced
Nopales, raw	0.015	1.16 cup sliced
Oranges, raw, Florida	0.015	.56 cup
Peaches, canned, juice pack, solids and liquids	0.015	.40 cup
Peaches, frozen, sliced, sweetened	0.015	.40 cup thawed
Squash, summer, scallop, cooked, boiled, drained, with salt	0.015	.48 cup
Squash, summer, scallop, cooked, boiled, drained, without salt	0.015	.48 cup
Squash, summer, zucchini, italian style, canned	0.015	.44 cup
Squash, winter, butternut, frozen, cooked, boiled, with salt	0.015	.48 cup
Squash, winter, butternut, frozen, cooked, boiled, without salt	0.015	.48 cup
Guavas, common, raw	0.016	.61 cup 1.8 fruit
Lettuce, green leaf, raw	0.016	2.78 cup shredded

Low Methionine Food List

Cure For The Garden: Featuring The Methionine Restriction Protocol   Copyright 2019. DocRhi.com

Lettuce, red leaf, raw	0.016	3.57 cup shredded .32 head
Nopales, cooked, without salt	0.016	.67 cup
Plums, dried (prunes), uncooked	0.016	.57 cup
Sesbania flower, raw	0.016	5 cup
Soymilk, original and vanilla, with added calcium, vitamins A and D	0.016	.41 cup
Squash, summer, zucchini, includes skin, frozen, cooked, boiled, drained, with salt	0.016	.45 cup
Squash, summer, zucchini, includes skin, frozen, cooked, boiled, drained, without salt	0.016	.45 cup
Asparagus, canned, no salt added, solids and liquids	0.017	.41 cup
Asparagus, canned, regular pack, solids and liquids	0.017	.41 cup
Bamboo shoots, cooked, boiled, drained, with salt	0.017	.83 cup sliced
Bamboo shoots, cooked, boiled, drained, without salt	0.017	.83 cup sliced
Beans, mung, mature seeds, sprouted, canned, drained solids	0.017	.80 cup
Carrots, cooked, boiled, drained, with salt	0.017	.64 cup
Carrots, cooked, boiled, drained, without salt	0.017	.64 cup
Dates, medjool	0.017	.53 cup 12 fruit
Grapes, canned, thompson seedless, water pack, solids and liquids	0.017	.41 cup
Okra, frozen, cooked, boiled, drained, without salt	0.017	.55 cup
Plantains, raw	0.017	.68 cup
Squash, summer, all varieties, raw	0.017	.88 cup
Squash, summer, scallop, raw	0.017	.77 cup sliced
Squash, summer, zucchini, includes skin, frozen, unprepared	0.017	.45 cup
Vegetables, mixed, canned, solids and liquids	0.017	
Beans, snap, green, frozen, cooked, boiled, drained without salt	0.018	.74 cup
Beans, snap, green, frozen, cooked, boiled, drained, with salt	0.018	.74 cup
Beans, snap, yellow, frozen, cooked, boiled, drained, with salt	0.018	.74 cup
Beans, snap, yellow, frozen, cooked, boiled, drained, without salt	0.018	.74 cup
Beet greens, raw	0.018	2.63 cup
Beets, raw	0.018	.74 cup
Cabbage, savoy, cooked, boiled, drained, with salt	0.018	.69 cup
Cabbage, savoy, cooked, boiled, drained, without salt	0.018	.69 cup
Kale, cooked, boiled, drained, with salt	0.018	.77 cup chopped
Kale, cooked, boiled, drained, without salt	0.018	.77 cup chopped
Kale, scotch, cooked, boiled, drained, with salt	0.018	.77 cup chopped
Kale, scotch, cooked, boiled, drained, without salt	0.018	.77 cup chopped
Leeks, (bulb and lower leaf-portion), raw	0.018	1.12 cup
Mountain yam, hawaii, raw	0.018	.74 cup .24 yam
Okra, frozen, cooked, boiled, drained, with salt	0.018	.55 cup
Okra, frozen, unprepared	0.018	1 cup
Pickle relish, hot dog	0.018	.41 cup
Squash, summer, crookneck and straightneck, frozen, cooked, boiled, drained, with salt	0.018	.52 cup
Squash, summer, crookneck and straightneck, frozen, cooked, boiled, drained, without salt	0.018	.52 cup
Squash, summer, zucchini, includes skin, raw	0.018	.88 sliced
Squash, winter, all varieties, raw	0.018	.71 cup cubes
Squash, winter, hubbard, baked, with salt	0.018	.49 cup
Squash, winter, hubbard, baked, without salt	0.018	.49 cup
Squash, winter, hubbard, cooked, boiled, mashed, with salt	0.018	.42 cup mashed
Squash, winter, hubbard, cooked, boiled, mashed, without salt	0.018	.42 cup mashed
Beets, cooked, boiled, drained	0.019	.59 cup

Cure For The Garden: Featuring The Methionine Restriction Protocol

Beets, cooked, boiled. drained, with salt	0.019	.59 cup
Chard, swiss, raw	0.019	2.8 cup
Hyacinth-beans, immature seeds, raw	0.019	1 1/4 cup
Mushrooms, canned, drained solids	0.019	.64 cup
Potatoes, canned, solids and liquids	0.019	.33 cup
Turnips, frozen, cooked, boiled, drained, with salt	0.019	.43 cup
Turnips, frozen, cooked, boiled, drained, without salt	0.019	.64 cup
Bamboo shoots, canned, drained solids	0.02	.76 cup
Cabbage, savoy, raw	0.02	1.4 cup shredded
Carrots, raw	0.02	.82 cup strips or sliced 1.6 medium
Cauliflower, raw	0.02	.93 cup chopped .17 head medium
Chard, swiss, cooked, boiled, drained, with salt	0.02	.57 cup
Chard, swiss, cooked, boiled, drained, without salt	0.02	.57 cup
Nuts, chestnuts, japanese, boiled and steamed	0.02	
Okra, cooked, boiled, drained, with salt	0.02	.63 cup
Okra, cooked, boiled, drained, without salt	0.02	.63 cup
Onions, spring or scallions (includes tops and bulb), raw	0.02	1 cup
Oranges, raw, all commercial varieties	0.02	.56 cup sections 1.04 small
Taro, raw	0.02	.96 cup
Watercress, raw	0.02	2.94 cup
Yam, cooked, boiled, drained, or baked, with salt	0.02	.74 cup
Yam, cooked, boiled, drained, or baked, without salt	0.02	.74 cup
Asparagus, canned, drained solids	0.021	.41 cup
Beet greens, cooked, boiled, drained, with salt	0.021	.69 cup 1" pieces
Beet greens, cooked, boiled, drained, without salt	0.021	.69 cup 1" pieces
Carambola, (starfruit), raw	0.021	.93 cup sliced 1.1 medium fruit
Cherimoya, raw	0.021	.63 cup
Grapes, american type (slip skin), raw	0.021	1.09 cup 42 fruit
Mustard greens, frozen, cooked, boiled, drained, with salt	0.021	.67 cup
Mustard greens, frozen, cooked, boiled, drained, without salt	0.021	.67 cup
Okra, raw	0.021	1 cup
Raisins, seedless	0.021	.61 cup packed
Yam, raw	0.021	
Beans, snap, green, frozen, all styles, microwaved	0.022	.74 cup
Beans, snap, green, frozen, all styles, unprepared	0.022	.74 cup
Beans, snap, green, raw	0.022	1 cup 1/2" pieces
Beans, snap, yellow, frozen, all styles, unprepared	0.022	.83 cup
Beans, snap, yellow, raw	0.022	1 cup 1/2 pieces
Dates, deglet noor	0.022	.68 cup
Lotus root, raw	0.022	.83 cup
Mushrooms, white, cooked, boiled, drained, with salt	0.022	.64 cup
Mushrooms, white, cooked, boiled, drained, without salt	0.022	.64 cup
Nuts, coconut cream, canned, sweetened	0.022	.34 cup
Oranges, raw, California, valencias	0.022	.56 cup
Pears, dried, sulfured, uncooked	0.022	.56 cup halves
Potatoes, canned, drained solids	0.022	.56 cup
Squash, winter, butternut, frozen, unprepared	0.022	.71 cup cubes
Coffee instant powder decaf	0.022	55 1/2 tsp
Beans, snap, green, cooked, boiled, drained, with salt	0.023	.8 cup
Beans, snap, green, cooked, boiled, drained, without salt	0.023	.80 cup

Low Methionine Food List

Cure For The Garden: Featuring The Methionine Restriction Protocol   Copyright 2019. DocRhi.com

178

Beans, snap, yellow, cooked, boiled, drained, with salt	0.023	.65 cup
Beans, snap, yellow, cooked, boiled, drained, without salt	0.023	.65 cup
Cauliflower, frozen, cooked, boiled, drained, with salt	0.023	.56 cup
Cauliflower, frozen, cooked, boiled, drained, without salt	0.023	.56 cup
Mountain yam, hawaii, cooked, steamed, with salt	0.023	.69 cup
Mountain yam, hawaii, cooked, steamed, without salt	0.023	.69 cup
Mustard greens, frozen, unprepared	0.023	.68 cup
Nuts, macadamia nuts, dry roasted, without salt added	0.023	.76 cup
Nuts, macadamia nuts, raw	0.023	.75 cup
Apricots, dehydrated (low-moisture), sulfured, uncooked	0.024	.40 cup 2/5 cup
Brussels sprouts, cooked, boiled, drained, with salt	0.024	.65 cup
Brussels sprouts, cooked, boiled, drained, without salt	0.024	.65 cup
Kiwifruit, green, raw	0.024	.56 cup sliced 1.45 fruit
Peppers, hot chili, green, raw	0.024	.67 cup
Peppers, hot chili, red, raw	0.024	.67 cup
Sapote, mamey, raw	0.024	.57 cup
Tomatoes, red, ripe, cooked, stewed	0.024	.99 cup
Mung beans, mature seeds, sprouted, cooked, boiled, drained, with salt	0.025	.81 cup
Mung beans, mature seeds, sprouted, cooked, boiled, drained, without salt	0.025	.81 cup
Mushrooms, shiitake, cooked, with salt	0.025	.69 cup
Mushrooms, shiitake, cooked, without salt	0.025	.69 cup
Seaweed, kelp, raw	0.025	1 1/4 cup
Squash, winter, hubbard, raw	0.025	.86 cup cubes
Sweet potato, cooked, boiled, without skin	0.025	.30 cup mashed
Cauliflower, cooked, boiled, drained, with salt	0.026	.81 cup
Cauliflower, cooked, boiled, drained, without salt	0.026	.81 cup
Hyacinth-beans, immature seeds, cooked, boiled, drained, with salt	0.026	1.15 cup
Hyacinth-beans, immature seeds, cooked, boiled, drained, without salt	0.026	1.15 cup
Kale, frozen, unprepared	0.026	.67 cup
Turnip greens, cooked, boiled, drained, with salt	0.026	.69 cup chopped
Turnip greens, cooked, boiled, drained, without salt	0.026	.69 cup chopped
Kale, frozen, cooked, boiled, drained, with salt	0.027	.77 cup chopped
Kale, frozen, cooked, boiled, drained, without salt	0.027	.77 cup chopped
Kale, scotch, raw	0.027	.67 cup
Oranges, raw, with peel	0.027	.59 cup
Potatoes, boiled, cooked without skin, flesh, with salt	0.027	.64 cup or .60 medium
Potatoes, boiled, cooked without skin, flesh, without salt	0.027	.64 cup or .60 medium
Shallots, raw	0.027	1 cup
Soymilk, original and vanilla, unfortified	0.027	.41 cup
Tomato products, canned, paste, without salt added	0.027	.43 cup
Asparagus, frozen, cooked, boiled, drained, with salt	0.028	.56 cup
Asparagus, frozen, cooked, boiled, drained, without salt	0.028	.56 cup
Cauliflower, frozen, unprepared	0.028	.76 cup
Collards, cooked, boiled, drained, with salt	0.028	.59 cup
Collards, cooked, boiled, drained, without salt	0.028	.59 cup
Peaches, dried, sulfured, stewed, without added sugar	0.028	.39 cup
Mushrooms, portabella, raw	0.029	.86 cup
Nuts, ginkgo nuts, canned	0.029	.65 cup 78 kernals
Sweet potato, raw, unprepared	0.029	.75 cup cubes
Bamboo shoots, raw	0.03	.66 cup
Mushrooms, enoki, raw	0.03	1.56 cup whole 33 1/3 fruit

Cure For The Garden: Featuring The Methionine Restriction Protocol   Copyright 2019. DocRhi.com

Low Methionine Food List

Potatoes, boiled, cooked in skin, flesh, with salt	0.03	.64 cup or .60 medium
Potatoes, boiled, cooked in skin, flesh, without salt	0.03	.64 cup or .60 medium
Sweet potato, canned, vacuum pack	0.03	.39 cup mashed
Swiss Chard	0.03	
Amaranth leaves, cooked, boiled, drained, with salt	0.031	.76 cup
Amaranth leaves, cooked, boiled, drained, without salt	0.031	.76 cup
Asparagus, frozen, unprepared	0.031	.56 cup
Asparagus, raw	0.031	.75 or 3/4 cup 6 1/4 spears medium
Mushrooms, white, raw	0.031	1.43 cup pieces
Peas and carrots, canned, no salt added, solids and liquids	0.031	.39 cup
Peas and carrots, canned, regular pack, solids and liquids	0.031	.39 cup
Potato puffs, frozen, unprepared	0.031	.83 cup
Potatoes, baked, flesh, with salt	0.031	.82 cup or 1/2 medium
Potatoes, baked, flesh, without salt	0.031	.82 cup or 1/2 medium
Seaweed, Canadian Cultivated EMI-TSUNOMATA, rehydrated	0.031	1 cup
Turnip greens, canned, solids and liquids	0.031	.43 cup
Vegetables, mixed, canned, drained solids	0.031	.61 cup
Brussels sprouts, raw	0.032	1.1 cup
Potatoes, flesh and skin, raw	0.032	.67 diced .47 medium
Potatoes, white, flesh and skin, baked	0.032	.67 cup
Collards, raw	0.033	2.8 cup
Collards, raw	0.033	2.8 cup
Mushrooms, shiitake, raw	0.033	.69 cup
Mushrooms, shiitake, stir-fried	0.033	.89 cup whole
Potatoes, microwaved, cooked in skin, flesh, with salt	0.033	.64 cup
Potatoes, microwaved, cooked in skin, flesh, without salt	0.033	.64 cup
Asparagus, cooked, boiled, drained	0.034	.56 cup
Asparagus, cooked, boiled, drained, with salt	0.034	.56 cup
Broccoli, flower clusters, raw	0.034	.71 cup
Broccoli, frozen, chopped, unprepared	0.034	.64 cup
Broccoli, stalks, raw	0.034	.66 cup, 3.23 spears
Figs, dried, uncooked	0.034	.67 cup
Jackfruit, raw	0.034	.66 cup 1" pieces
Mung beans, mature seeds, sprouted, raw	0.034	.96 cup
Mushrooms, white, stir-fried	0.034	.93 cup
Potato puffs, frozen, oven-heated	0.034	.78 cup 14 1/4 puffs
Turnip greens, raw	0.034	1.82 cup chopped
Vegetables, mixed, frozen, cooked, boiled, drained, with salt	0.034	.55 cup
Vegetables, mixed, frozen, cooked, boiled, drained, without salt	0.034	.55 cup
Brussels sprouts, frozen, cooked, boiled, drained, with salt	0.035	.65 cup
Brussels sprouts, frozen, cooked, boiled, drained, without salt	0.035	.65 cup
Dock, raw	0.035	.75 chopped
Mushrooms, portabella, grilled	0.035	.83 cup
Potatoes, red, flesh and skin, baked	0.035	.67 cup diced or .47 medium
Seeds, breadnut tree seeds, raw	0.035	
Swamp cabbage (skunk cabbage), cooked, boiled, drained, without salt	0.035	1.78 cup
Swamp cabbage (skunk cabbage), cooked, boiled, drained, with salt	0.035	1.78 cup
Amaranth leaves, raw	0.036	3.6 cups
Basil, fresh	0.036	4.2 cup whole leaf
Brussels sprouts, frozen, unprepared	0.036	1.1 cup
Chives, raw	0.036	100 tsp

Cure For The Garden: Featuring The Methionine Restriction Protocol   Copyright 2019. DocRhi.com

Yardlong bean, cooked, boiled, drained, with salt	0.036	.96 cup slices
Yardlong bean, cooked, boiled, drained, without salt	0.036	.96 slices
Avocados, raw, California	0.037	.43 cup
Broccoli, frozen, chopped, cooked, boiled, drained, with salt	0.037	.54 cup
Broccoli, frozen, chopped, cooked, boiled, drained, without salt	0.037	.54 cup
Broccoli, frozen, spears, cooked, boiled, drained, with salt	0.037	.55 cup
Broccoli, frozen, spears, cooked, boiled, drained, without salt	0.037	.55 cup
Broccoli, frozen, spears, unprepared	0.037	.64 cup
Collards, frozen, chopped, unprepared	0.037	2.8 cup
Lambsquarters, cooked, boiled, drained, with salt	0.037	.56 cup
Lambsquarters, cooked, boiled, drained, without salt	0.037	.56 cup
Peas and onions, frozen, cooked, boiled, drained, with salt	0.037	.56 cup
Peas and onions, frozen, cooked, boiled, drained, without salt	0.037	.56 cup
Sweet potato, cooked, baked in skin, flesh, with salt	0.037	.50 cup
Sweet potato, cooked, baked in skin, flesh, without salt	0.037	.50 cup
Avocados, raw, all commercial varieties	0.038	.43 cup pureed, 1/2 fruit
Broccoli, raw	0.038	1.1 cup
Mushrooms, portabella, exposed to ultraviolet light, grilled	0.038	.83 cup
Nuts, chestnuts, european, raw, peeled	0.038	.70 cup
Nuts, chestnuts, european, raw, peeled	0.038	.70 cup
Nuts, coconut milk, canned (liquid expressed from grated meat and water)	0.038	.44 cup
Nuts, coconut milk, canned (liquid expressed from grated meat and water)	0.038	.44 cup
Potatoes, baked, flesh and skin, with salt	0.038	.82 cup or 1/2 medium
Potatoes, baked, flesh and skin, without salt	0.038	.82 cup or 1/2 medium
Potatoes, frozen, whole, unprepared	0.038	.78 cup
Avocado	0.038	
Potatoes, microwaved, cooked in skin, flesh and skin, without salt	0.039	.64 cup
Potatoes, microwaved, cooked, in skin, flesh and skin, with salt	0.039	.64 cup
Spinach, canned, no salt added, solids and liquids	0.039	.43 cup
Spinach, canned, regular pack, solids and liquids	0.039	.43 cup
Squash, zucchini, baby, raw	0.039	.81 cup
Collards, frozen, chopped, cooked, boiled, drained, with salt	0.04	.59 cup
Collards, frozen, chopped, cooked, boiled, drained, without salt	0.04	.59 cup
Lima beans, immature seeds, canned, no salt added, solids and liquids	0.04	.42 cup
Lima beans, immature seeds, canned, regular pack, solids and liquids	0.04	.42 cup
Vegetables, mixed, frozen, unprepared	0.04	
Yardlong bean, raw	0.04	1.1 cup sliced
Okara	0.041	.82 cup
Sweet potato, cooked, boiled, without skin, with salt	0.041	.30 cup mashed
Avocados, raw, Florida	0.042	.43 cup
Cauliflower, green, raw	0.042	1.56 cup .23 head medium
Cowpeas (blackeyes), immature seeds, raw	0.042	.69 cup
Hearts of palm, canned	0.042	.68 cup
Litchis, dried	0.042	
Mushrooms, oyster, raw	0.042	1.16 cup sliced
Parsley, fresh	0.042	1.67 cup
Sweet potato, frozen, cooked, baked, with salt	0.042	.57 cup cubes
Sweet potato, frozen, cooked, baked, without salt	0.042	.57 cup cubes
Sweet potato, frozen, unprepared	0.042	.57 cup
Broadbeans, immature seeds, raw	0.043	.92 cup

Cure For The Garden: Featuring The Methionine Restriction Protocol   Copyright 2019. DocRhi.com

Broccoli, cooked, boiled, drained, with salt	0.043	.78 cup
Broccoli, cooked, boiled, drained, without salt	0.043	.78 cup
Cauliflower, green, cooked, no salt added	0.043	.8 cup
Cauliflower, green, cooked, with salt	0.043	.8 cup
Nuts, coconut milk, raw (liquid expressed from grated meat and water)	0.043	.42 cup
Taro leaves, cooked, steamed, without salt	0.043	.69 cup
Taro, leaves, cooked, steamed, with salt	0.043	.69 cup
Buckwheat, whole groat flour	0.043	
Beans, kidney, mature seeds, sprouted, raw	0.044	.54 cup
Peas and carrots, frozen, cooked, boiled, drained, with salt	0.044	.63 cup
Potatoes, french fried, all types, salt added in processing, frozen, home-prepared, oven heated	0.044	.47 cup
Swamp cabbage, (skunk cabbage), raw	0.044	1.79 cup chopped
Broadbeans (fava beans), mature seeds, canned	0.045	.39 cup
Cowpeas (blackeyes), immature seeds, cooked, boiled, drained, with salt	0.045	.61 cup
Cowpeas (blackeyes), immature seeds, cooked, boiled, drained, without salt	0.045	.61 cup
Peas and carrots, frozen, cooked, boiled, drained, without salt	0.045	.63 cup
Spearmint, fresh	0.046	4 cups
Peas, green, canned, regular pack, solids and liquids	0.047	.40 cup
Peas, green, canned, seasoned, solids and liquids	0.047	.40 cup
Potatoes, hash brown, home-prepared	0.047	.64 cup
Pumpkin leaves, cooked, boiled, drained, with salt	0.047	1.41 cup
Pumpkin leaves, cooked, boiled, drained, without salt	0.047	1.41 cup
Rosemary, fresh	0.047	58.8 Tbsp
Broccoli raab, raw	0.048	2.5 cup
Mushrooms, brown, italian, or crimini, raw	0.048	1.15 cup
Mushrooms, portabella, exposed to ultraviolet light, raw	0.048	.86 cup
Peaches, dehydrated (low-moisture), sulfured, stewed	0.048	.41 cup
Peas and onions, canned, solids and liquids	0.048	.83 cup
Peas, green, canned, no salt added, solids and liquids	0.048	.40 cup
Turnip greens and turnips, frozen, unprepared	0.048	
Longans, dried	0.049	
Peas and carrots, frozen, unprepared	0.049	.72 cup
Sweet potato, canned, mashed	0.049	.39 cup mashed
Seeds, breadnut tree seeds, dried	0.05	
Sweet potato leaves, cooked, steamed, with salt	0.05	1.56 cup
Sweet potato leaves, cooked, steamed, without salt	0.05	1.56 cup
Jute, potherb, cooked, boiled, drained, with salt	0.051	1.15 cup
Jute, potherb, cooked, boiled, drained, without salt	0.051	1.15 cup
Spinach, canned, regular pack, drained solids	0.052	.43 cup
Spinach, frozen, chopped or leaf, unprepared	0.052	.64 cup
Mung beans, mature seeds, sprouted, cooked, stir-fried	0.053	.96 cup
Peppermint, fresh	0.053	4 cups
Spinach, frozen, chopped or leaf, cooked, boiled, drained, with salt	0.053	.53 cup
Spinach, frozen, chopped or leaf, cooked, boiled, drained, without salt	0.053	.53 cup
Spinach, raw	0.053	3 1/3 cup
Nuts, chestnuts, japanese, raw	0.054	
Pumpkin leaves, raw	0.054	2.56 cup
Nuts, ginkgo nuts, raw	0.055	78 kernals
Spinach, cooked, boiled, drained, with salt	0.055	.56 cup

Cure For The Garden: Featuring The Methionine Restriction Protocol   Copyright 2019. DocRhi.com

Low Methionine Food List

Spinach, cooked, boiled, drained, without salt	0.055	.56 cup
Beans, pinto, mature seeds, canned, solids and liquids	0.056	.58 cup
Beans, pinto, mature seeds, canned, solids and liquids, low sodium	0.056	.58 cup
Carrot, dehydrated	0.056	1.35 cup
Turnip greens, frozen, unprepared	0.056	1.82 cup chopped
Broccoli raab, cooked	0.058	2.5 cup
Peas and onions, frozen, unprepared	0.059	.73 cup
Lima beans, immature seeds, frozen, fordhook, cooked, boiled, drained, with salt	0.06	.59 cup
Lima beans, immature seeds, frozen, fordhook, cooked, boiled, drained, without salt	0.06	.59 cup
Broadbeans (fava beans), mature seeds, cooked, boiled, with salt	0.062	.59 cup
Broadbeans (fava beans), mature seeds, cooked, boiled, without salt	0.062	.59 cup
Lima beans, large, mature seeds, canned	0.062	.41 cup
Nuts, coconut meat, raw	0.062	1.3 cup
Lima beans, immature seeds, frozen, fordhook, unprepared	0.063	.64 cup
Seaweed, wakame, raw	0.063	1 1/4 cup
Beans, navy, mature seeds, sprouted, raw	0.064	.96 cup
Chickpeas (garbanzo beans, bengal gram), mature seeds, canned, solids and liquids	0.065	.42 cup
Chickpeas (garbanzo beans, bengal gram), mature seeds, canned, solids and liquids, low sodium	0.065	.42 cup
Hyacinth beans, mature seeds, cooked, boiled, with salt	0.065	.52 cup
Hyacinth beans, mature seeds, cooked, boiled, without salt	0.065	.52 cup
Jute, potherb, raw	0.065	3.57 cup
Refried beans, canned, traditional, reduced sodium	0.065	.42 cup
Turnip greens and turnips, frozen, cooked, boiled, drained, with salt	0.065	.61 cup
Turnip greens and turnips, frozen, cooked, boiled, drained, without salt	0.065	.61 cup
Lima beans, immature seeds, frozen, baby, cooked, boiled, drained, with salt	0.066	.56 cup
Lima beans, immature seeds, frozen, baby, cooked, boiled, drained, without salt	0.066	.56 cup
Cowpeas, common (blackeyes, crowder, southern), mature seeds, canned, plain	0.067	.58 cup
Peas, green, canned, no salt added, drained solids	0.067	.40 cup
Peas, green, canned, no salt added, drained solids	0.067	.40 cup
Beans, kidney, all types, mature seeds, canned	0.068	.39 cup
Lima beans, immature seeds, cooked, boiled, drained, with salt	0.068	.59 cup
Lima beans, immature seeds, cooked, boiled, drained, without salt	0.068	.59 cup
Lima beans, immature seeds, cooked, boiled, drained, without salt	0.068	.59 cup
Lima beans, immature seeds, raw	0.068	.64 cup
Nuts, coconut cream, raw (liquid expressed from grated meat)	0.068	.42 cup
Peas, green (includes baby and lesuer types), canned, drained solids, unprepared	0.068	.57 cup
Peas, green (includes baby and lesuer types), canned, drained solids, unprepared	0.068	.57 cup
Drumstick leaves, cooked, boiled, drained, with salt	0.069	.42 cup
Drumstick leaves, cooked, boiled, drained, without salt	0.069	.42 cup
Peas, mature seeds, sprouted, raw	0.069	.83 cup
Peas, mature seeds, sprouted, raw	0.069	.83 cup
Seeds, breadfruit seeds, boiled	0.069	
Beans, kidney, red, mature seeds, canned, solids and liquid, low sodium	0.07	.39 cup
Beans, kidney, red, mature seeds, canned, solids and liquids	0.07	.39 cup

Cure For The Garden: Featuring The Methionine Restriction Protocol   Copyright 2019. DocRhi.com

Nuts, chestnuts, chinese, boiled and steamed	0.07	.65 cup
Nuts, chestnuts, japanese, roasted	0.071	.65 cup
Seeds, lotus seeds, raw	0.072	3.13 cup
Bananas, dehydrated, or banana powder	0.074	1 cup
MORI-NU, Tofu, silken, soft	0.074	3.5 oz
Onions, dehydrated flakes	0.074	1.8 cup
Lima beans, immature seeds, frozen, baby, unprepared	0.075	.61 cup
Mothbeans, mature seeds, cooked, boiled, with salt	0.075	.56 cup
Mothbeans, mature seeds, cooked, boiled, without salt	0.075	.56 cup
Nuts, chestnuts, european, roasted	0.075	.65 cup
Radishes, oriental, dried	0.075	.86 cup
Garlic, raw	0.076	.74 cup
Mustard, prepared, yellow	0.076	.40 cup
Pigeon peas (red gram), mature seeds, cooked, boiled, with salt	0.076	.60 cup
Pigeon peas (red gram), mature seeds, cooked, boiled, without salt	0.076	.60 cup
Turnip greens, frozen, cooked, boiled, drained, with salt	0.076	.61 cup
Turnip greens, frozen, cooked, boiled, drained, without salt	0.076	.61 cup
Lentils, mature seeds, cooked, boiled, with salt	0.077	.51 cup
Lentils, mature seeds, cooked, boiled, without salt	0.077	.51 cup
MORI-NU, Tofu, silken, lite firm	0.077	3.5 oz
Peas, green, frozen, cooked, boiled, drained, with salt	0.078	.63 cup
Peas, green, frozen, cooked, boiled, drained, without salt	0.078	.63 cup
Spices, cinnamon, ground	0.078	38.5 tsp
Beans, adzuki, mature seed, cooked, boiled, with salt	0.079	.43 cup
Beans, adzuki, mature seeds, cooked, boiled, without salt	0.079	.43 cup
Beans, black turtle, mature seeds, canned	0.079	.42 cup
Beans, black, mature seeds, canned, low sodium	0.079	.42 cup
Peas, green, frozen, unprepared	0.079	.75 cup
Taro leaves, raw	0.079	3.57 cup
Hummus, home prepared	0.08	.41 cup
Spices, cloves, ground	0.08	47.62 tsp
Carob flour	0.081	.97 cup
Peas, green, cooked, boiled, drained, with salt	0.081	.63 cup
Peas, green, cooked, boiled, drained, without salt	0.081	.63 cup
Seeds, breadfruit seeds, roasted	0.081	
Peas, green, raw	0.082	.69 cup
Beans, cranberry (roman), mature seeds, canned	0.083	.38 cup
Refried beans, canned, traditional style (includes USDA commodity)	0.083	.23 cup
Mung beans, mature seeds, cooked, boiled, with salt	0.084	.50 cup
Mung beans, mature seeds, cooked, boiled, without salt	0.084	.50 cup
Tofu, soft, prepared with calcium sulfate and magnesium chloride (nigari)	0.084	3.5 oz
Beans, pinto, canned, drained solids	0.085	.59 cup
Peas, split, mature seeds, cooked, boiled, with salt	0.085	.51 cup
Peas, split, mature seeds, cooked, boiled, without salt	0.085	.51 cup
Beans, pinto, mature seeds, canned, drained solids, rinsed in tap water	0.086	.59 cup
Sweet potato leaves, raw	0.086	2.86 cup chopped
Goji berries, dried	0.087	.91 cup
Peaches, dried, sulfured, uncooked	0.087	.63 cup
MORI-NU, Tofu, silken, lite extra firm	0.088	3.5 oz
Soybeans, mature seeds, sprouted, cooked, steamed	0.089	1.06 cup
Soybeans, mature seeds, sprouted, cooked, steamed, with salt	0.089	1.06 cup

Cure For The Garden: Featuring The Methionine Restriction Protocol   Copyright 2019. DocRhi.com

Low Methionine Food List

184

Spices, ginger, ground	0.089	19.23 tbsp
Spices, onion powder	0.09	.91 cup
Chickpeas (garbanzo beans, bengal gram), mature seeds, canned, drained solids	0.093	.66 cup
Chickpeas (garbanzo beans, bengal gram), mature seeds, canned, drained, rinsed in tap water	0.093	.66 cup
MORI-NU, Tofu, silken, extra firm	0.094	3.5 oz
Beans, great northern, mature seeds, canned	0.096	.38 cup
Beans, great northern, mature seeds, canned, low sodium	0.096	.38 cup
Seeds, breadfruit seeds, raw	0.096	.45 cup
Spices, pepper, black	0.096	55 1/2 tsp
Beans, navy, mature seeds, canned	0.098	.55 cup
Lima beans, large, mature seeds, cooked, boiled, with salt	0.099	.56 cup
Lima beans, large, mature seeds, cooked, boiled, without salt	0.099	.56 cup
Nuts, coconut meat, dried (desiccated), creamed	0.099	1.1 cup
Nuts, coconut meat, dried (desiccated), toasted	0.099	1.1 cup
Peas, green, canned, drained solids, rinsed in tap water	0.1	.61 cup
Nuts, chestnuts, chinese, raw	0.101	.65 cup
Lima beans, thin seeded (baby), mature seeds, cooked, boiled, with salt	0.102	.55 cup
Lima beans, thin seeded (baby), mature seeds, cooked, boiled, without salt	0.102	.55 cup
Nuts, acorns, raw	0.103	
Beans, kidney, red, mature seeds, canned, drained solids	0.104	.56 cup
Tofu, salted and fermented (fuyu)	0.104	.40 cup
Lentils, sprouted, raw	0.105	1.3 cup
Beans, french, mature seeds, cooked, boiled, with salt	0.106	.56 cup
Beans, french, mature seeds, cooked, boiled, without salt	0.106	.56 cup
Beans, kidney, red, mature seeds, canned, drained solids, rinsed in tap water	0.106	.63 cup
MORI-NU, Tofu, silken, firm	0.106	3.5 oz
Potato flour	0.107	.63 cup
Nuts, chestnuts, chinese, roasted	0.108	.65 cup
Tofu, raw, regular, prepared with calcium sulfate	0.108	.40 cup
Beans, white, mature seeds, canned	0.109	.38 cup
Tofu, salted and fermented (fuyu), prepared with calcium sulfate	0.109	.40 cup
Winged beans, mature seeds, cooked, boiled, with salt	0.109	.38 cup
Winged beans, mature seeds, cooked, boiled, without salt	0.109	.38 cup
Cowpeas, common (blackeyes, crowder, southern), mature seeds, cooked, boiled, with salt	0.11	.58 cup
Cowpeas, common (blackeyes, crowder, southern), mature seeds, cooked, boiled, without salt	0.11	.58 cup
Lupins, mature seeds, cooked, boiled, with salt	0.11	.60 cup
Lupins, mature seeds, cooked, boiled, without salt	0.11	.60 cup
Mung beans, mature seeds, cooked, boiled, with salt	0.11	.56 cup
Mung beans, mature seeds, cooked, boiled, without salt	0.11	.56 cup
Tofu, firm, prepared with calcium sulfate and magnesium chloride (nigari)	0.11	.40 cup
Beans, navy, mature seeds, cooked, boiled, with salt	0.111	.55 cup
Beans, navy, mature seeds, cooked, boiled, without salt	0.111	.55 cup
Spices, garlic powder	0.111	10 1/3 tbsp
Beans, kidney, all types, mature seeds, cooked, boiled, without salt	0.113	.56 cup
Chickpeas (garbanzo beans, bengal gram), mature seeds, cooked, boiled, with salt	0.116	.61 cup

Cure For The Garden: Featuring The Methionine Restriction Protocol   Copyright 2019. DocRhi.com

Chickpeas (garbanzo beans, bengal gram), mature seeds, cooked, boiled, without salt	0.116	.61 cup
Cowpeas, catjang, mature seeds, cooked, boiled, with salt	0.116	.58 cup
Cowpeas, catjang, mature seeds, cooked, boiled, without salt	0.116	.58 cup
Beans, pinto, mature seeds, cooked, boiled, without salt	0.117	.58 cup
Nuts, chestnuts, european, boiled and steamed	0.118	.70 cup
Peaches, dehydrated (low-moisture), sulfured, uncooked	0.118	.86 cup
Yardlong beans, mature seeds, cooked, boiled, with salt	0.118	.58 cup
Yardlong beans, mature seeds, cooked, boiled, without salt	0.118	.58 cup
Miso	0.12	.36 cup 5.88 Tbsp
Cowpeas (blackeyes), immature seeds, frozen, cooked, boiled, drained, with salt	0.121	.59 cup
Cowpeas (blackeyes), immature seeds, frozen, cooked, boiled, drained, without salt	0.121	.59 cup
Nuts, almond butter, plain, with salt added	0.122	.40 cup
Nuts, almond butter, plain, without salt added	0.122	.40 cup
Tofu, extra firm, prepared with nigari	0.122	3.5 oz
Tomatoes, sun-dried	0.122	1.85 cup
Tomatoes, sun-dried	0.122	1.85 cup
Beans, black turtle, mature seeds, cooked, boiled, with salt	0.123	.54 cup
Beans, black turtle, mature seeds, cooked, boiled, without salt	0.123	.54 cup
Drumstick leaves, raw	0.123	.21 cup
Beans, great northern, mature seeds, cooked, boiled, with salt	0.125	.56 cupp
Beans, great northern, mature seeds, cooked, boiled, without salt	0.125	.56 cup
Beans, pinto, mature seeds, cooked, boiled, with salt	0.126	.58 cup
Nuts, acorn flour, full fat	0.126	
Nuts, chestnuts, japanese, dried	0.126	.65 cup
Peppers, hot chile, sun-dried	0.127	.37 cup
Spices, oregano, dried	0.127	33 1/3 tbsp or 100 tsp
Cowpeas (blackeyes), immature seeds, frozen, unprepared	0.128	.63 cup
Miso	0.129	.36 cup
Nuts, coconut meat, dried (desiccated), not sweetened	0.129	1.08 cup shredded
Nuts, coconut meat, dried (desiccated), not sweetened	0.129	1.08 cup shredded
Beans, kidney, all types, mature seeds, cooked, boiled, with salt	0.13	.56 cup
Beans, kidney, red, mature seeds, cooked, boiled, with salt	0.13	.56 cup
Beans, kidney, red, mature seeds, cooked, boiled, without salt	0.13	.56 cup
Spices, chili powder	0.13	12 1/2 tbsp
Beans, black, mature seeds, cooked, boiled, with salt	0.133	.58 cup
Beans, black, mature seeds, cooked, boiled, without salt	0.133	.58 cup
Edamame, frozen, unprepared	0.133	.85 cup
Frijoles rojos volteados (Refried beans, red, canned)	0.133	.43 cup
Nuts, ginkgo nuts, dried	0.133	78 kernals
Shallots, freeze-dried	0.134	6.9 cup
Beans, small white, mature seeds, cooked, boiled, with salt	0.135	.56 cup
Beans, small white, mature seeds, cooked, boiled, without salt	0.135	.56 cup
Beans, pink, mature seeds, cooked, boiled, with salt	0.136	.59 cup
Beans, pink, mature seeds, cooked, boiled, without salt	0.136	.59 cup
Nuts, acorns, dried	0.136	
Beans, kidney, california red, mature seeds, cooked, boiled, with salt	0.137	.56 cup
Beans, kidney, california red, mature seeds, cooked, boiled, without salt	0.137	.56 cup
Beans, yellow, mature seeds, cooked, boiled, with salt	0.138	.56 cup
Beans, yellow, mature seeds, cooked, boiled, without salt	0.138	.56 cup

Cure For The Garden: Featuring The Methionine Restriction Protocol   Copyright 2019. DocRhi.com

Soybeans, mature seeds, sprouted, raw	0.138	1.43 cup
Soybeans, mature seeds, sprouted, raw	0.138	1.43 cup
Beans, cranberry (roman), mature seeds, cooked, boiled, with salt	0.14	.56 cup
Beans, cranberry (roman), mature seeds, cooked, boiled, without salt	0.14	.56 cup
Spices, turmeric, ground	0.14	11 1/3tbsp or 33.33 tsp
Edamame, frozen, prepared	0.141	.65 cup
Peppers, ancho, dried	0.142	5.9 peppers
Beans, kidney, royal red, mature seeds, cooked, boiled with salt	0.143	.56 cup
Beans, kidney, royal red, mature seeds, cooked, boiled, without salt	0.143	.56 cup
Spices, dill seed	0.143	11 1/4 cup
Seaweed, laver, raw	0.145	38 sheets
Beans, white, mature seeds, cooked, boiled, with salt	0.146	.53 cup large
Beans, white, mature seeds, cooked, boiled, without salt	0.146	.53 cup large
Nuts, beechnuts, dried	0.146	
Soybeans, green, cooked, boiled, drained, with salt	0.15	.56 cup
Soybeans, green, cooked, boiled, drained, without salt	0.15	.56 cup
Nuts, chestnuts, european, dried, unpeeled	0.151	.65 cup
Nuts, almonds, dry roasted, with salt added	0.155	.70 cup
Nuts, almonds, dry roasted, without salt added	0.155	.70 cup
Nuts, almonds	0.157	.70 whole 1.09 sliced 1.05 ground
Soybeans, green, raw	0.157	.39 cup
Nuts, chestnuts, chinese, dried	0.165	1.1 cup flour
Peanuts, all types, cooked, boiled, with salt	0.166	.56 cup
Soy sauce made from soy (tamari)	0.167	.38 cup
Tofu, hard, prepared with nigari	0.169	.40 cup cubed
Tempeh	0.175	.60 cup
Mushrooms, shiitake, dried	0.179	5 1/4 whole
Leeks, (bulb and lower-leaf portion), freeze-dried	0.18	31 1/4 cup
Nuts, pecans	0.183	.73 cup
Nuts, pecans, oil roasted, with salt added	0.183	.73 cup
Nuts, pecans, oil roasted, without salt added	0.183	.73 cup
Falafel, home-prepared	0.187	depends on ingredients and size
Nuts, almonds, oil roasted, lightly salted	0.188	.73 cup
Nuts, almonds, oil roasted, with salt added	0.188	.73 cup
Nuts, almonds, oil roasted, without salt added	0.188	.73 cup
Nuts, pecans, dry roasted, with salt added	0.189	.73 cup
Nuts, pecans, dry roasted, without salt added	0.189	.73 cup
Nuts, almonds, blanched	0.19	.69 cup
Spices, curry powder	0.19	15.9 tbsp
Hyacinth beans, mature seeds, raw	0.191	.48 cup
Spices, paprika	0.2	14.7 tbsp
Cocoa unsweetened powder	0.202	.85 cup 40 1/2 tsp
Nuts, hazelnuts or filberts, blanched	0.203	1.33 ground .74 whole
Nuts, cashew butter, plain, with salt added	0.204	.73 cup
Nuts, pine nuts, pinyon, dried	0.207	.74 cup
Natto	0.208	.57 cup
Beans, adzuki, mature seeds, raw	0.21	.51 cup
Beans, adzuki, mature seeds, raw	0.21	.51 cup
Lentils, raw	0.21	.52 cup
Parsley, freeze-dried	0.21	17 3/4 cup
Tofu, raw, firm, prepared with calcium sulfate	0.211	.40 cup

Cure For The Garden: Featuring The Methionine Restriction Protocol   Copyright 2019. DocRhi.com

Lentils, pink or red, raw	0.212	.52 cup
Broadbeans (fava beans), mature seeds, raw	0.213	.67 cup
Peppers, sweet, green, freeze-dried	0.215	15 3/4 cup
Peppers, sweet, red, freeze-dried	0.215	15 3/4 cup
Mothbeans, mature seeds, raw	0.22	.51 cup
Tofu, fried	0.22	.40 cubes
Nuts, hazelnuts or filberts	0.221	.74 whole .87 chopped 71 nuts
Nuts, hazelnuts or filberts, dry roasted, without salt added	0.222	.63 cup
Soybeans, mature cooked, boiled, without salt	0.224	.58 cup
Soybeans, mature seeds, cooked, boiled, with salt	0.224	.58 cup
Nuts, mixed nuts, dry roasted, with peanuts, with salt added	0.228	.73 cup
Tofu, fried, prepared with calcium sulfate	0.23	.40 cubes
Chives, freeze-dried	0.231	31 cup
Nuts, walnuts, english	0.236	.85 cup
Pigeon peas (red gram), mature seeds, raw	0.243	.49 cup
Peas, green, split, mature seeds, raw	0.251	.51 cup
Sausage, meatless	0.253	depends on brand
Seaweed, Canadian Cultivated EMI-TSUNOMATA, dry	0.254	5 cup
Lupins, mature seeds, raw	0.255	.56 cup
Beans, pinto, mature seeds, raw	0.259	.52 cup
Nuts, pine nuts, dried	0.259	.74 cup
Nuts, mixed nuts, dry roasted, with peanuts, without salt added	0.26	.73 cup
Lima beans, thin seeded (baby), mature seeds, raw	0.261	.50 cup
Peanut butter, chunk style, with salt	0.262	.39 cup
Peanut butter, chunk style, without salt	0.262	.39 cup
USDA Commodity, Peanut Butter, smooth	0.262	.39 cup
Peanut butter, smooth style, with salt	0.265	.39 cup
Peanut butter, smooth style, without salt	0.265	.39 cup
Seeds, lotus seeds, dried	0.267	3.13 cup
Chickpeas (garbanzo beans, bengal gram), mature seeds, raw	0.27	.50 cup
Lima beans, large, mature seeds, raw	0.271	.56 cup
Beans, navy, mature seeds, raw	0.273	.48 cup
Nuts, cashew nuts, dry roasted, with salt added	0.274	.73 cup
Nuts, cashew nuts, dry roasted, without salt added	0.274	.73 cup
Spearmint, dried	0.281	
Beans, french, mature seeds, raw	0.283	.54 cup
Nuts, mixed nuts, oil roasted, with peanuts, lightly salted	0.283	.73 cup
Nuts, mixed nuts, oil roasted, with peanuts, with salt added	0.283	.73 cup
Nuts, mixed nuts, oil roasted, with peanuts, without salt added	0.283	.73 cup
Seeds, safflower seed kernels, dried	0.284	
Mung beans, mature seeds, raw	0.286	.48 cup
Peanuts, all types, dry-roasted, with salt	0.291	.68 cup
Peanuts, all types, dry-roasted, without salt	0.291	.68 cup
Peanuts, all types, oil-roasted, with salt	0.291	.68 cup
Peanuts, all types, oil-roasted, without salt	0.291	.68 cup
Veggie burgers or soyburgers, unprepared	0.291	depends on brand
Nuts, hickorynuts, dried	0.3	.83 cup
Spices, fennel seed	0.301	50 tsp or 19.9 tbsp
Peanuts, valencia, raw	0.308	.68 cup
Peanuts, virginia, raw	0.309	.68 cup
Seeds, sisymbrium sp. seeds, whole, dried	0.311	1.35 cup
Beans, pink, mature seeds, raw	0.315	.48 cup

Low Methionine Food List

Cure For The Garden: Featuring The Methionine Restriction Protocol   Copyright 2019. DocRhi.com

Nuts, cashew butter, plain, without salt added	0.315	.73 cup
Beans, small white, mature seeds, raw	0.317	.47 cup
Peanuts, all types, raw	0.317	.68 cup
Peanuts, virginia, oil-roasted, with salt	0.317	.70 cup
Peanuts, virginia, oil-roasted, without salt	0.317	.70 cup
Beans, black turtle, mature seeds, raw	0.32	.54 cup
Spices, basil, dried	0.32	22.2 tbsp
Nuts, mixed nuts, oil roasted, without peanuts, lightly salted	0.321	.69 cup
Peanuts, spanish, raw	0.321	.68 cup
Beans, black, mature seeds, raw	0.325	.58 cup
Beans, great northern, mature seeds, raw	0.329	.55 cup
Beans, yellow, mature seeds, raw	0.331	.51 cup
Peanuts, valencia, oil-roasted, with salt	0.332	.69 cup
Peanuts, valencia, oil-roasted, without salt	0.332	.69 cup
Nuts, cashew nuts, oil roasted, with salt added	0.334	.78 cup whole or halves
Nuts, cashew nuts, oil roasted, without salt added	0.334	.78 cup whole or halves
Cowpeas, common (blackeyes, crowder, southern), mature seeds, raw	0.335	.42 cup
Spices, fenugreek seed	0.338	27 tsp or 9 tbsp
Beans, kidney, red, mature seeds, raw	0.339	.54 cup
Cowpeas, catjang, mature seeds, raw	0.34	.60 cup
Peanuts, spanish, oil-roasted, with salt	0.344	.68 cup
Peanuts, spanish, oil-roasted, without salt	0.344	.68 cup
Beans, cranberry (roman), mature seeds, raw	0.346	.51 cup
Nuts, mixed nuts, oil roasted, without peanuts, with salt added	0.346	.69 cup
Nuts, mixed nuts, oil roasted, without peanuts, without salt added	0.346	.69 cup
Yardlong beans, mature seeds, raw	0.346	.60 or 3/5 cup
Yardlong beans, mature seeds, raw	0.346	.60 or 3/5 cup
Beans, white, mature seeds, raw	0.351	.47 cup small
Beans, kidney, all types, mature seeds, raw	0.355	.54 cup
Winged beans, mature seeds, raw	0.356	.55 cup
Nuts, pistachio nuts, raw	0.36	.81 cup
Spices, caraway seed	0.361	.93 cup
Nuts, cashew nuts, raw	0.362	.73 cup
Beans, kidney, california red, mature seeds, raw	0.367	.54 cup
Seeds, flaxseed	0.37	.60 or 3/5 cup whole 14.3 tbsp ground
Seeds, sunflower seed kernels, toasted, with salt added	0.374	.75 cup
Seeds, sunflower seed kernels, toasted, without salt	0.374	.75 cup
Nuts, pistachio nuts, dry roasted, with salt added	0.375	.81 cup
Nuts, pistachio nuts, dry roasted, without salt added	0.375	.81 cup
Beans, kidney, royal red, mature seeds, raw	0.381	.54 cup
Nuts, pilinuts, dried	0.395	.83 cup
Peanut flour, low fat	0.415	1.67 cup
Seeds, pumpkin and squash seeds, whole, roasted, with salt added	0.417	1.56 cup
Seeds, pumpkin and squash seeds, whole, roasted, without salt	0.417	1.56 cup
Seeds, sunflower seed kernels from shell, dry roasted, with salt added	0.42	.78 cup
Seeds, sunflower seed kernels, dry roasted, with salt added	0.42	.78 cup
Seeds, sunflower seed kernels, dry roasted, without salt	0.42	.78 cup
Palo Verdi seeds immature	0.43	
Seeds, sunflower seed butter, with salt added	0.435	6 1/4 tbsp
Seeds, sunflower seed butter, without salt	0.435	6 1/4 tbsp
Seeds, sunflower seed kernels, oil roasted, with salt added	0.435	.74 cup

Cure For The Garden: Featuring The Methionine Restriction Protocol　　　Copyright 2019. DocRhi.com

Seeds, sunflower seed kernels, oil roasted, without salt	0.435	.74 cup
Soy flour, full-fat, raw	0.466	1.19 cup
Nuts, walnuts, black, dried	0.467	.80 cup
Soy flour, full-fat, roasted	0.469	1.18 cup
Soybeans, mature seeds, roasted, no salt added	0.475	.58 cup
Soybeans, mature seeds, roasted, salted	0.475	.58 cup
Spices, mustard seed, ground	0.483	15.87 tbsp
Seeds, sunflower seed kernels, dried	0.494	.78 cup
Spices, poppy seed	0.502	11 1/3 tbsp
Seeds, cottonseed kernels, roasted (glandless)	0.529	.67 cup
Soybeans, mature seeds, dry roasted	0.534	1 cup
Soybeans, mature seeds, raw	0.547	.54 cup
Seeds, sesame meal, partially defatted	0.56	1.56 cup
Seeds, sesame seed kernels, toasted, with salt added (decorticated)	0.56	.67 cup
Seeds, sesame seed kernels, toasted, without salt added (decorticated)	0.56	.67 cup
Seeds, sesame seeds, whole, roasted and toasted	0.56	.69 cup
Seeds, sesame butter, tahini, from roasted and toasted kernels (most common type)	0.561	6 2/3 cup
Seeds, sesame seeds, whole, dried	0.586	.69 cup
Seeds, chia seeds, dried	0.588	.63 cup
Seeds, sesame butter, tahini, from raw and stone ground kernels	0.588	6 2/3 tbsp
Seeds, sesame butter, tahini, from unroasted kernels (non-chemically removed seed coat)	0.593	6 2/3 tbsp
Seeds, pumpkin and squash seed kernels, roasted, with salt added	0.595	.85 cup
Seeds, pumpkin and squash seed kernels, roasted, without salt	0.595	.85 cup
Spices, parsley, dried	0.596	62 1/2 tbsp
Seeds, sesame butter, paste	0.597	6 2/3 tbsp
Seeds, pumpkin and squash seed kernels, dried	0.603	.78 cup
Soy meal, defatted, raw	0.606	.82 cup
Nuts, butternuts, dried	0.611	.83 cup
Tofu, dried-frozen (koyadofu)	0.613	.40 cup
Tofu, dried-frozen (koyadofu), prepared with calcium sulfate	0.613	.40 cup
Seeds, safflower seed meal, partially defatted	0.625	
Soy flour, defatted	0.634	.95 cup
Peanut flour, defatted	0.641	.60 cup
Seeds, watermelon seed kernels, dried	0.834	.93 cup
Seeds, sesame seed kernels, dried (decorticated)	0.88	.67 cup
Palo Verdi seeds	0.88	
Seeds, hemp seed, hulled	0.933	.62 cup
Seeds, sesame flour, high-fat	1.016	.67 cup
Seeds, sunflower seed flour, partially defatted	1.043	1.56 cup
Nuts, brazilnuts, dried, unblanched	1.124	.75 cup
Soy protein isolate	1.13	.58 cup
Soy protein isolate, potassium type	1.13	.58 cup
Seaweed, spirulina, dried	1.149	.89 cup
Seeds, sesame flour, partially defatted	1.331	.16 cup
Seeds, sesame flour, low-fat	1.656	.67 cup
FOOD	100g	AMOUNT OF FOOD
FOODS (grams of methionine in 100 grams of food)	/100 g	Volume of food
Methionine measurements found at Dept. of Agriculture website		
Amount of food in 100g found at traditionaloven.com or		

Cure For The Garden: Featuring The Methionine Restriction Protocol   Copyright 2019. DocRhi.com

Supplemental Reading

Orgeron, M. et al. (2014) The Impact of Dietary Methionine Restriction on Biomarkers of Metabolic Health. Prog Mol Biol Transl Sci.; 121: 351–376. doi:10.1016/B978-0-12-800101-1.00011-9

Plaisance, E. et al, (2011) Dietary Methionine Restriction Increases Fat Oxidation in Obese Adults with Metabolic Syndrome The Journal of Clinical Endocrinology & Metabolism 96:5, E836-E840. DOI: http://dx.doi.org/10.1210/jc.2010-2493

Clinton, C. et al (2015) Whole-Foods, Plant-Based Diet Alleviates the Symptoms of Osteoarthritis. Arthritis. Article ID 708152, 9 pages. http://dx.doi.org/10.1155/2015/708152

Watanabe, F. et al.. (2014). Vitamin B12-Containing Plant Food Sources for Vegetarians. Nutrients, 6(5), 1861–1873. http://doi.org/10.3390/nu6051861

Rajdl, D. (2016) Effect of Folic Acid, Betaine, Vitamin B_6, and Vitamin B12 on Homocysteine and Dimethylglycine Levels in Middle-Aged Men Drinking White Wine.. Nutrients. Jan 12;8(1). pii: E34. doi: 10.3390/nu8010034.

Giannella, R. et al. (1971). Vitamin B12 uptake by intestinal microorganisms: mechanism and relevance to syndromes of intestinal bacterial overgrowth. Journal of Clinical Investigation, 50(5), 1100–1107.

Desiree et al (2014)Transcriptional Impact of Dietary Methionine Restriction on Systemic Inflammation: Relevance to Biomarkers of Metabolic, Disease During Aging.. Biofactors. January ; 40(1): 13–26. doi:10.1002/biof.1111.

Mozafar, A. Plant Soil (1994) 167: 305. doi:10.1007/BF00007957
James, M. et al (2008) Effects of Food Natural Products on the Biotransformation of PCBs. Environ Toxicol Pharmacol. March ; 25(2): 211–217

Plaisance, E. (2011) Dietary Methionine Restriction Increases Fat Oxidation in Obese Adults with Metabolic Syndrome. Jounal of Clinical Endocrinology & Metabolism. Vol. 96:5. DOI: http://dx.doi.org/10.1210/jc.2010-2493

Supplemental Reading

Fraser, G. (1999), Associations Between Diet and Cancer, Ischemic Heart Disease, and All-Cause Mortality in Non-Hispanic White California Seventh-day Adventists. Am J Clin Nutr September 1999 vol. 70 no. 3 532s-538s, http://ajcn.nutrition.org/content/70/3/532s.full

Vazquez-Marti, A. et al.(2012)Phenolic Secoiridoids in Extra Virgin Olive Oil Impede Fibrogenic and Oncogenic Epithelial-to-Mesenchymal Transition: Extra Virgin Olive Oil As a Source of Novel Antiaging Phytochemicals REJUVENATION RESEARCH Volume 15, Number 1. DOI: 10.1089/rej.2011.1203 source PubMed. https://www.researchgate.net/publication/221733242

Lees, E. et al (2014) Methionine restriction restores a younger metabolic phenotype in adult mice with alterations in fibroblast growth factor 21. Aging Cell 13, pp817–827. Doi: 10.1111/acel.12238

Johnson, J. et al. (2014) Methionine Restriction Activates the Retrograde Response and Confers Both Stress Tolerance and Lifespan Extension to Yeast, Mouse and Human Cells. PLoS One. 2014; 9(5): e97729. Published online May 15. doi: 10.1371/journal.pone.0097729

Salim, Samina. (2014). Oxidative Stress and Psychological Disorders, Current Neuropharmacology, 2014, 12, 140-147. doi: 10.2174/1570159X11666131120230309

Longo, V. et al. (2015) Interventions to Slow Aging in Humans: Are We Ready? Aging Cell 14, pp497–510, doi: 10.1111/acel.12338

Sugimbra, T, et al. Quantitative nutritional studies with water-soluble, chemically defined diets. 8. The forced feeding of diets each lacking in one essential amino acid. Lab. Biochem., Nat. Cancer Inst., Bethesda, Md. Archives of Biochemistry. 1959. Vol.81 pp.448-455

Cooke D1, Ouattara A1, Ables Dietary methionine restriction modulates renal response and attenuates kidney injury in mice. GP1. FASEB J. 2017 Sep 28:fj201700419R. doi: 10.1096/fj.201700419R.

Cheril Tapia-Rojas, et al. "Is L-methionine a trigger factor for Alzheimer's-like neurodegeneration?: Changes in Aβ oligomers, tau phosphorylation, synaptic proteins, Wnt signaling and behavioral impairment in wild-type mice." Mol Neurodegener. 2015; 10: 62. doi: 10.1186/s13024-015-0057-0

Supplemental Reading

Methionine restriction leads to Aβ reduction and neuroprotection: Implications in Alzheimer's disease pathogenesis and prevention July 2015. Volume 11, Issue 7, Supplement, Pages P838–P839

Koichi Hirabayashi, et al. Neurologically normal development of a patient with severe methionine adenosyl transferase I/III deficiency after continuing dietary methionine restriction. Gene. Volume 530, Issue 1, 1 November 2013, Pages 104-108 https://doi.org/10.1016/j.gene.2013.08.025

Gharibzadeh S. Et al. Depression and fruit treatment. J Neuropsychiatry Clin Neurosci. 2010 Fall;22(4):451-m.e25-451.e25. doi: 10.1176/appi.neuropsych.22.4.451-m.e25.

Disclaimer

DISCLAIMER: THIS BOOk DOES NOT PROVIDE MEDICAL ADVICE
The information, including but not limited to, text, graphics, images and other material contained in this book are for informational purposes only. The purpose of this book is to promote broad consumer understanding and knowledge of various health topics. It is not intended to be a substitute for professional medical advice, diagnosis or treatment. Always seek the advice of your physician or other qualified health care provider with any questions you may have regarding a medical condition or treatment and before undertaking a new health care regimen, and never disregard professional medical advice or delay in seeking it because of something you have read on this website. It does not recommend or endorse any specific tests, physicians, products, procedures, opinions or other information that may be mentioned on this website. Reliance on any information appearing in this book is solely at your own risk.

Made in the USA
Monee, IL
30 July 2021